BABY BOOT CAMP

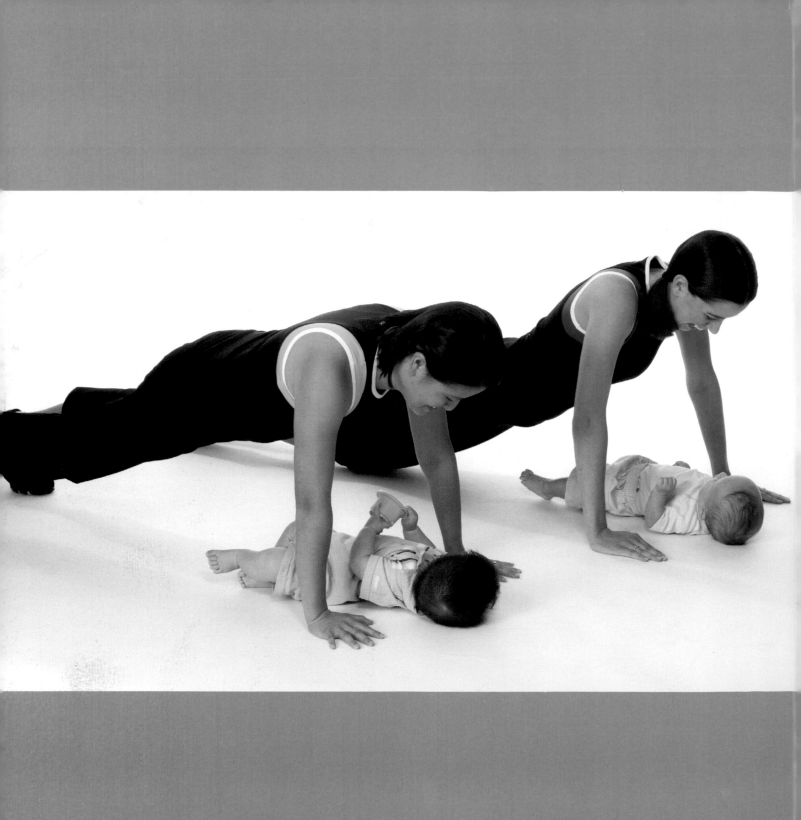

BABY BOOT CAMP

The New Mom's 9-Minute Fitness Solution

Kristen Horler, CEO & Founder of Baby Boot Camp®

with Amanda Vogel

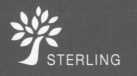

STERLING

New York / London
www.sterlingpublishing.com

Library of Congress Cataloging-in-Publication Data
Horler, Kristen with Vogel, Amanda.
  Baby boot camp : the new mom's 9-minute fitness solution/Kristen Horler
with Amanda Vogel.
      p. cm.
  Includes index.
  ISBN 978-1-4027-5873-7
1. Exercise for women. 2. Physical fitness for women. 3. Mothers—Health and
hygiene. 4. Postnatal care. I. Title. II. Title: New mom's nine-minute fitness
solution.

GV482.H67 2010
613.71082—dc22

      2009006851

10 9 8 7 6 5 4 3 2 1

Published by Sterling Publishing Co., Inc.
387 Park Avenue South, New York, NY 10016
© 2009 by Baby Boot Camp LLC
Distributed in Canada by Sterling Publishing
$^{C}/_{O}$ Canadian Manda Group, 165 Dufferin Street
Toronto, Ontario, Canada M6K 3H6
Distributed in the United Kingdom by GMC Distribution Services
Castle Place, 166 High Street, Lewes, East Sussex, England BN7 1XU
Distributed in Australia by Capricorn Link (Australia) Pty. Ltd.
P.O. Box 704, Windsor, NSW 2756, Australia

Book design and layout: *tabula rasa* graphic design

Printed in China
All rights reserved

Sterling ISBN 978-1-4027-5873-7

For information about custom editions, special sales, premium and corporate purchases, please contact Sterling Special Sales Department at
800-805-5489 or specialsales@sterlingpublishing.com.

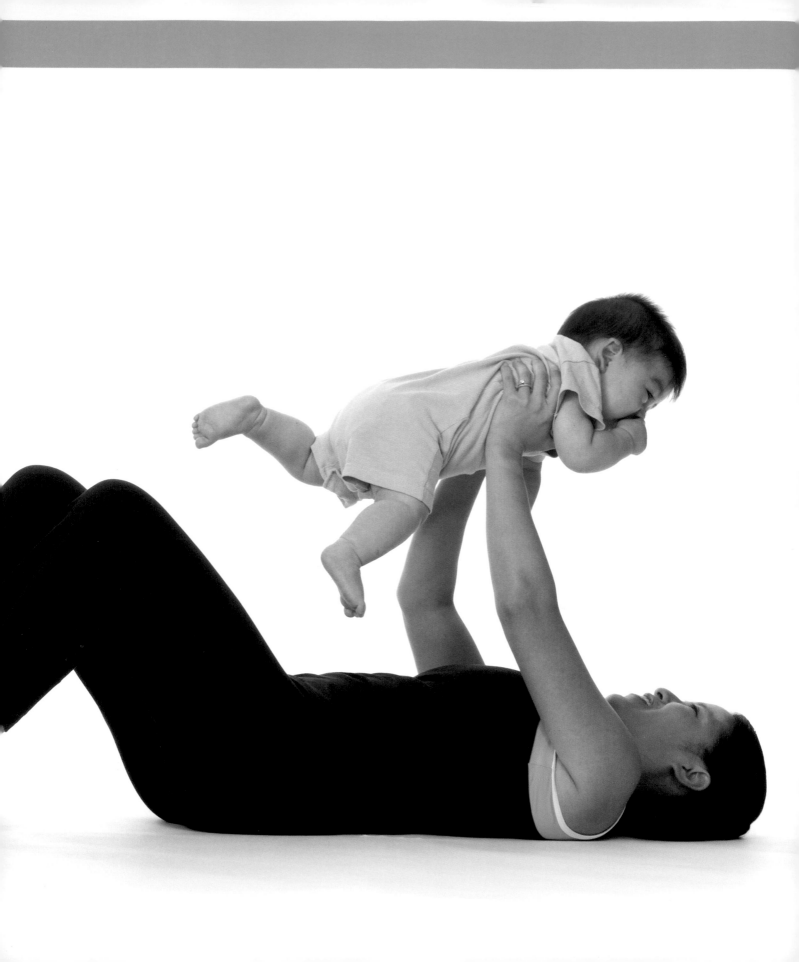

CONTENTS

As the founder and CEO of Baby Boot Camp, I am inspired every day by new moms just like you—and the thousands of women who participate in and teach Baby Boot Camp classes every week. Through them (and my own experiences as a mom), I have learned what is most realistic when it comes to exercising with a baby (or two) in tow. For nearly a decade, one of my life goals was to write a fitness book to meet the needs of new moms. I am thrilled that, with the help of my team, I have now made it a reality!

I first started Baby Boot Camp to help moms enjoy the many benefits of getting and staying fit—together. One of Baby Boot Camp's key goals is to provide safe and effective workouts for *real moms*. It's now my pleasure to share my proven and successful program with you, in the form of this book, to enable you to exercise in the comfort of your home.

An active lifestyle is one of the greatest gifts you can share with your children, and I sincerely hope the exercises, tips, and encouragement I have included in this book will inspire you to make physical activity part of each day. There's no time like the present to get started with exercise, so turn the page and let's go!

Love,
Kristen

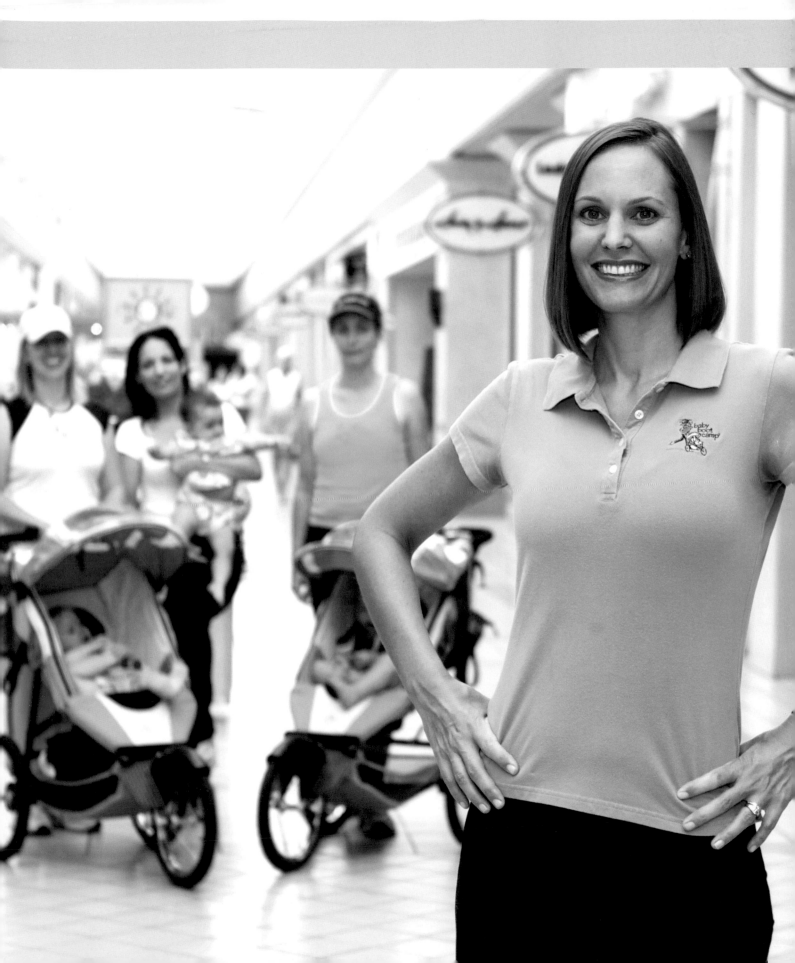

t's been 18 years since I had my last child, and 24 years since I had my first. When I was home with my children, connecting with friends often involved a pot of coffee and a box of 24-count donuts. Although getting together with other mothers was vital to my mental health, it wasn't doing a whole lot for my physical health.

For years, exercise was perceived as an activity only for athletes or for those with extra time on their hands. However, study after study has shown that exercise greatly helps with depression. And although exercise for new mothers was unheard of thirty or forty years ago, today we know the important role it plays not only in mental recovery but physical recovery as well.

I don't think I am alone in experiencing the challenges of coming home with a new baby, especially when it's your fourth. It was only because I had kept my body active with my last two pregnancies that I was able not only to experience a great, healthy pregnancy and delivery, but a quick post-partum recovery with enhanced energy and a strong body.

The demands of motherhood—at all stages—makes regular exercise absolutely vital in our daily routine. However, for many moms, everyone else comes first and, more often than not, exercise falls to the bottom of the list. Women are amazing in their ability to multitask and take on what would be for others, i.e. men, an insurmountable list of daily to-do's. Yet most mothers don't blink an eye and effortlessly carry out each task. However, as our children get older, the stress of everyday life and demands starts to take a toll on our bodies. Therefore, we know that exercising during and after pregnancy is not only the best thing women can do, it's essential.

After reading through Kristen's book, my first thought was, "As a young mother, I would have given a million dollars to have a resource like this!" So many moms put pressure on themselves to make exercise an all-day project when the reality is time is of the essence when you have children. Kristen clearly understands the stress and time issues mothers deal with every day and beautifully addresses them in checklists and time management suggestions throughout the book. A 25-year fitness veteran and mother, she is keenly aware that a little bit of something is a whole lot better than a lot of nothing, and reminds new mothers to be patient with the process of getting their bodies back to pre-baby size. Her personal parenting experiences and the day-to-day challenges mothers face are all meticulously covered in *Baby Boot Camp: The New Mom's 9-minute Fitness Solution.*

For years I have tried to explain the importance of time efficiency to the mothers I work with, and this book provides time-efficient exercises. So leave behind the guilt of not going to a club for two hours a day. *Baby Boot Camp* provides a great option to the stress that going to a gym typically serves up. The reality is that for many moms exercise is lost if a child is sick or time is usurped in a doctor's office. But Kristen's book helps you realize that exercise, even though brief, can be effective.

Many other books offer "generic" programming that rarely addresses specifics for individual needs. *Baby Boot Camp* makes finding appropriate exercises easy and, most importantly, user appropriate. In addition to the specific exercise chapters, based on fitness level, Kristen also thoughtfully addresses the physical aches and pains during and after pregnancy.

Baby Boot Camp will not only find a permanent spot wherever you choose to work out, it is an ideal gift for any expecting or new mother. Kristen's relaxed tone and easy-to-understand information, tips, and exercises make this book a must for all new mothers. There is no better time for women to be educated in healthy living, not only for themselves but also for their children. *Baby Boot Camp* is a brilliant resource for moms and a solid health and fitness resource for their families.

Here's to Healthy Families!

—Nicki Anderson,
   president of Reality Fitness, Inc.

   2008/2009 IDEA Personal Trainer of the Year

   Author of *Reality Fitness: Inspiration for Your Health and Well-Being*

INTRODUCTION Welcome to Baby Boot Camp!

I am excited to have this opportunity to share the benefits of improved health and fitness with you while you enjoy spending valuable time bonding with your baby. This book covers the first twelve months of your journey with your new baby. During this time, your beautiful baby will change in so many amazing ways . . . and so will your postpregnancy body!

Consider this book your survival guide to the physical changes that come with your new life. It's quite natural for your body to be in a state of flux right now. What your physique looks like this week might be very different from what it looked like in the days after giving birth or from the body you'll see in the mirror just a few weeks from now.

Getting Your Prebaby Body Back

Whether you've just had your first baby or you've experienced the postpartum phase of motherhood before, you're probably reading this book for solutions to a common concern of any new mom: Getting your prebaby body back as soon as possible. After nine months of maternity clothes and weight gain, you're ready to shed pounds and shape up. The dilemma is this: Who has time for exercise with a newborn to care for? You do!

The exercises in this book are packaged in such a way that squeezing an entire routine into your tiring and time-crunched day is actually possible. There's no assumption that you have up to an hour to spare per workout (and that your baby will cooperate for that duration). The Baby Boot Camp at-home workouts in this book are quick—just nine minutes long—so you can do them before baby's short attention span and fussing lead

to tossing in the towel on fitness. And since you've probably come to cherish any activity that entertains your baby while also giving you a chance to energize yourself, you'll appreciate how most of the moves can be done while you cuddle or interact with your newborn.

Nine minutes is all you need (plus a few extra moments for warm-up and stretching). Of course, you have the option to exercise more as you start to feel stronger and your baby's mood and age allow for slightly longer exercise/playtimes. But whether you do just one nine-minute routine or squeeze in a couple at a time (or throughout your day), you'll get a well-rounded workout for your abs, back, legs, butt, shoulders, and arms. Through the mom-friendly and baby-friendly exercises, you will learn how to improve your strength, relieve aches and pains, look better, feel better, and be the best mom you can be (even when you are sleep-deprived).

Every chapter includes a routine you can do using just your body weight and/or your baby as resistance. Some chapters include an additional routine that incorporates hand weights to help you achieve noticeable results more quickly. It's time to get your body back in shape! I'll show you how to do it within your limited time and with your limited energy.

Be Fit. Be Strong. Be Together.

Integrating a fitness plan into your life after having a baby is a juggling act I understand well because I have two young kids of my own. As a mom, I know firsthand how tough it is to get, well, *anything* done with one or more babies in tow. After my first child was born in 2001, I was anxious to start feeling stronger and to lose the sixty-five pregnancy pounds I'd gained. Yet I was torn between wanting my prepregnancy shape back and the unappealing prospect of having to hire a babysitter or leave my newborn with strangers at the gym.

I tried a few fitness videos at home, but they didn't solve the problem of how to keep my baby entertained, and, as a certified personal trainer with the American Council on Exercise (ACE), I knew that the videos' exercises weren't always appropriate for my postnatal body. The weather in San Francisco, where I lived at the time, made stroller-walking a decent option. Still, doing just that every day lacked variety—for a well-rounded fitness program, I knew I needed strength and flexibility training, too, not just cardio.

Like most new moms, I wanted to nurture and bond with my baby as much as possible. So I rounded up a small group of women whose goals, like mine, were to get fit, connect with other new parents, and, most importantly, find an activity their babies would also benefit from and have fun doing.

We met in a local park twice a week and worked out together with our babies. Every week, those three women came back with stories of moms they'd spoken to who wanted "in" on our workouts. Soon, I started receiving requests for more classes, at more locations, on more days a week. This is how my company, Baby Boot Camp—now a fast-growing international franchise for prenatal and postpartum fitness—was born. The company's tagline is *Be fit. Be strong. Be together.*® I hope it's the experience you will gain from this book as well.

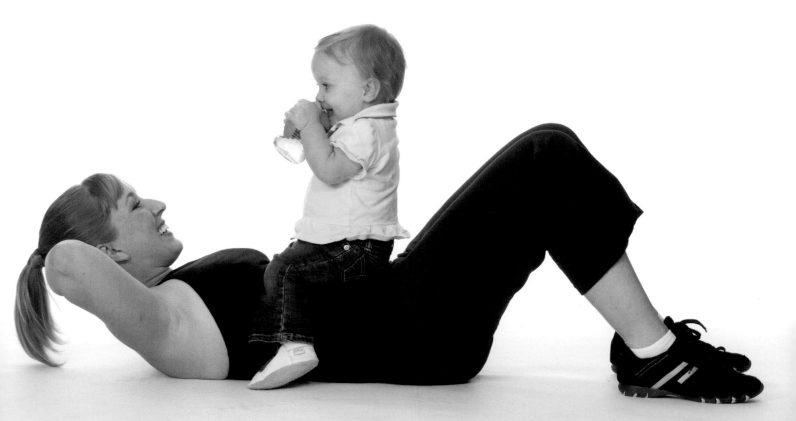

HOW TO USE THIS BOOK

Like the thousands of women worldwide who now join Baby Boot Camp classes every week, you're probably hoping your body bounces back sooner rather than later. You might be focused on shrinking the extra skin and extra weight you see in the mirror. You can reach that goal with the exercises in this book, which are specifically geared to your postpartum body. Remember, though, that exercise in the postnatal months requires the same care as exercise during pregnancy. You're not pregnant anymore, but your body is still in flux. Believe it or not, successfully improving what you see on the *outside* means giving your body time to heal on the *inside*. The exercises on the pages to come take into account how issues such as loose joints, weak abs and back, postural changes, and the birth experience affect which postnatal exercises you can and should do. You'll also find exercise modifications for women who've delivered by C-section.

Look at it this way: It takes *nine* months and *three* trimesters for your body to undergo incredible change as it nurtures a new life. The following chapters will help you return to your prebaby shape (or better!) *nine* minutes at a time, *three* days a week. And since getting back in shape after having a baby—or at any time, for that matter—is a process, I've organized this book so you can read it in very manageable chunks.

How to Get Started

Most other postpartum exercise books require time-starved moms like you to read lots of chapters—or the entire book—to learn the exercise concepts before you can kick off a fitness program. I don't know about you, but when I had my first baby, I barely had time to read the cooking instructions on a package of frozen lasagna, let alone an entire book about fitness! With that in mind, I wrote *Baby Boot Camp* so it's easy for you to get started right away. All you have to do is read one exercise chapter at a time, much like the format of those baby guides you're poring over these days. Have you noticed how baby books for new parents usually allow you to read in short spurts, so you get just the need-to-know info for your baby's age as it is right now? That's what this book is modeled after. Simply read the exercise chapter that matches your baby's age, follow the exercise routines on those pages, and save the rest for later! You'll get to tackle the exercises in easy-to-handle blocks of time, so you won't ever feel overwhelmed by too many choices or guilty that you haven't been able to get started because you're still wading through pages of explanations.

As a bonus, you'll feel a sense of accomplishment as you "complete" each chapter and progress to new moves. And since each chapter corresponds to your baby's age, you'll get motivation from seeing how your baby's age-related milestones complement the exercises. For example, each exercise chapter begins with a place to record your baby's weight, so you can compare how much more you're lifting over time—an indication that you're getting stronger. Each exercise also contains a Trainer Tip to help you get the most out an exercise and avoid injury. And look for my Intensity Tips, which describe how to make an exercise harder once you've become familiar with it. Remember: The more you challenge yourself, the faster you'll start to see results.

So let me guide you through the three components of fitness taught in Baby Boot Camp classes: cardio, stretching, and strength training. In the chapters that follow, you'll find step-by-step, calorie-burning cardio workouts you can do outdoors while baby rides along in the stroller. Chapter 7 shows you the best mom-and-baby stretches for limbering up muscles that get especially tight from tasks like breast- or bottle-feeding and stooping over during diaper changes. The main focus of this book, however, complements Baby Boot Camp's signature format: strength training. These are the nine-minute routines. Since this is the first book to offer a whole-body, at-home strength-training program that changes with your baby's age and developmental stages, I explain in chapter 1 why strength training is so important in the early stages of motherhood.

IT'S NEVER TOO LATE TO GET STARTED

If you happen to be reading this book after your baby is no longer a newborn, it's not too late to get started!

• If you don't do any strength training now, start with the exercises in chapter 3, even though your baby is older. Do those moves for about four weeks, then move on to chapter 4, following the guidelines you'll find there.

• If you've been doing one to three days of strength training already (including for your core, back, and pelvic floor—see the three key postpartum exercises in chapter 3, pages 22 and 23) and your baby is more than twelve weeks old, go on to chapter 4 now.

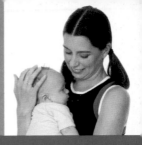

PART 1

Why New Moms Need Strength Training

CHAPTER 1

It's Not Just about "Baby Fat"

Although it's true that most new moms rank weight loss at the top of their wish lists for getting back in shape after having a baby, they'll also tell you it's not just about melting away the "baby fat." As a woman in the postpartum phase—what some experts call the fourth trimester—you're experiencing many physical and emotional changes as well.

For example, sleep deprivation could be affecting your energy levels right now. (Granted, this book won't make your baby sleep longer, but the exercises can make you feel more alert.) You might be dealing with back pain and discomfort from postural changes that occurred during pregnancy and the demands you're under these days. You may be experiencing incontinence—that is, uncontrolled leaking of urine. If you're nursing, your breasts might feel tender. Even your joints are more loose and less stable than normal—a by-product of breast-feeding and/or your recent pregnancy. And that's just the physical stuff! On the emotional side, you may be grappling with body image issues, feelings of depression and guilt, or anxiety about doing anything for yourself (such as exercise). So, you see, feeling and looking better—or "getting your body back"—extends well beyond a concern about

losing unwanted pounds. And that's where strength training fits in.

What Strength Training Can Do for You Right Now

As the months pass after your delivery, your body will slowly return to its prepregnancy state, or close to it anyway. Still, what you do now can help that process along and ensure that you bounce back in the best way possible, with greater ease, less pain and discomfort, and more confidence about how you look. Here are three major benefits of strength training for new moms.

1. Strength Training Reduces Your Risk of Injury

Meeting an infant's constant needs is challenging enough without also nursing an injury, especially one that could have been avoided. Truth is, you need muscle to safely handle the demands of being a new mom. Sure, your baby might be relatively light now (if you're reading this shortly after your little one was born). But most babies double their birth weight by five or six months and triple it by a year. You might be faring OK with eight or ten pounds (3.6–4.5kg) these days, but are you ready for sixteen or twenty pounds (7.3–9kg) in a few months? Will you be able to safely lift and carry a young toddler who's twenty-five or thirty pounds (11.4–13.6kg)?

Apart from picking up and holding your growing baby, you're probably lugging around an awkward car seat, lifting a stroller in and out of the back of your vehicle, and slinging a stuffed diaper bag over your shoulder wherever you go. And you're performing all these mommy duties while you're recovering from being pregnant and delivering a baby! It's no wonder that you're particularly susceptible right now to aggravating old injuries or developing new ones. Strength training—even just a few days a week—will help stave off injury by creating stronger muscles all over your body, including those that surround injury-prone joints.

2. Strength Training Eases Common Postpartum Discomforts

You've just experienced nine months of body-altering pregnancy and delivering a baby (by birth canal or C-section), and now you're functioning on little sleep while managing around-the-clock parenting duties. Chances are, you're facing one or more common postpregnancy discomforts, such as neck aches, backaches, sore wrists, and more. Fortunately, the right strengthening and stretching exercises can help.

- *Your neck and shoulders.* Even the tiniest baby can start to feel like a heavy load after you've been carrying her in a front carrier or sling for more than ten or fifteen minutes. The result is sore, burning muscles, particularly around your shoulders and neck. Use the upper-body strengthening exercises throughout this book to boost strength around your shoulder joints and spine—doing so will make activities such as carrying your baby and all her gear feel much more comfortable. Refer to pages 114 and 116 for stretches that counteract tightness in the neck and shoulder area.

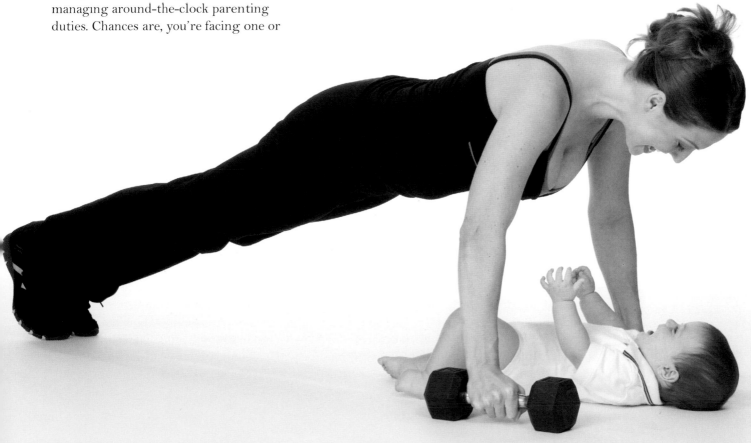

- **Your back.** Considering that 50–90 percent of women report back discomfort during pregnancy, it stands to reason that this discomfort would persist postpregnancy. Strengthening your abdominals and back muscles with the right postpartum exercises helps lessen or prevent pain and discomfort caused by everything from postural misalignments that developed when you were expecting to carrying around extra pregnancy pounds, to slouching forward during diaper changes or baby feedings, to the effects of weak, overstretched abs. Simply put, the stronger you make all your muscles—especially your abs and lower back—the less strain you'll feel from day-to-day activities.

- **Your wrists.** More than a quarter of expecting women experience carpal tunnel syndrome due to fluid retention and pregnancy-related changes in the joints. These symptoms can persist or even crop up for the first time in the postpartum phase, and, unfortunately, tasks like breast-feeding or bottle-feeding, stroller-walking, carrying a car seat, and even the way you hold your baby can make matters worse. While you must avoid certain exercises if you do have carpal tunnel syndrome, you can help prevent this problem from occurring in the first place by strengthening the muscles around your wrists and in your arms.

- **Your hips and thighs.** You might experience discomfort from compression on the sciatic nerve, which feels like a shooting pain in the hip and down one leg. As a postpartum woman, you're especially prone to sciatic pain because of postural imbalances from pregnancy and habits you may have formed now in the postpartum stage, such as always holding your baby on the same side of your body. In the next chapter, I'll show you how to start alleviating this pesky postpartum-related pain.

- **Your knees.** It's not uncommon for women who've had a baby to complain of knee pain. One reason is because of the hormone relaxin, which peaks in the first trimester and again just before you deliver. Its job is to make your joints looser and less stable, which aids with labor and delivery. However, relaxin sticks around for about three months after delivery, or for as long as you breast-feed, which explains why it might be aggravating your knees now. Although strength training doesn't change the presence or levels of relaxin in your body, it can help alleviate other sources of knee discomfort, such as imbalances in the legs due to certain muscles being weak and overstretched while opposing ones are strong and tight. Muscle imbalances like this can occur from pregnancy-related postural changes and/or all that sitting you're doing these days as your newborn enjoys drawn-out feeds at the breast or with a bottle.

3. Strength Training Boosts Your Body Image

It's no secret that any amount of exercise makes you feel almost instantly better about how you look. This can have a positive impact on your self-confidence, and not just in terms of body image. Mentally, you feel more confident about your abilities to carry out activities like collapsing a stubborn stroller or scooping up a squirming one-year-old without tweaking something in your back. If you're experiencing incontinence, you may feel comforted to know that the pelvic-floor strengthening exercises (Kegels) found in this book (see page 22)

can help reduce or alleviate the problem—
another confidence booster.

Plus, as a nice bonus, having more lean
body mass (muscle) from doing resistance
exercise allows you to burn more calories at
work, at play, and even during rest periods.
The more calories you comfortably and
safely burn each day, the faster you'll lose
unwanted pregnancy pounds.

Baby Boot Camp Basics

Now that you've read about some of the
benefits of strength training in the postpartum phase, I hope you're ready to launch a
program of your own. Before you do,
however, please review the tips below for
working out with hand weights or using
your baby or your own body weight as
resistance. Finally, use the checklist at the
end of this chapter to ensure that every
workout you do with your baby goes as
smoothly as possible for both of you.

• Maintain slow, controlled movements. Of
  course, when you lift your baby during
  an exercise, you'll naturally move slowly
  and with good control. It's your mother's
  instinct! Take that same approach when
  using hand weights: Lift dumbbells for
  two counts and lower them for two counts
  on each repetition.

• Breathe out through your mouth on the
  effort of lifting the hand weights or your
  baby. Breathe in through your nose as you
  lower the resistance.

• Use dumbbells between five and ten
  pounds (2.3–4.5kg) for the hand weight
  routines in this book. When you can
  easily lift a dumbbell for three sets of
  forty-five seconds each, it's time to select
  heavier hand weights. As for your baby's

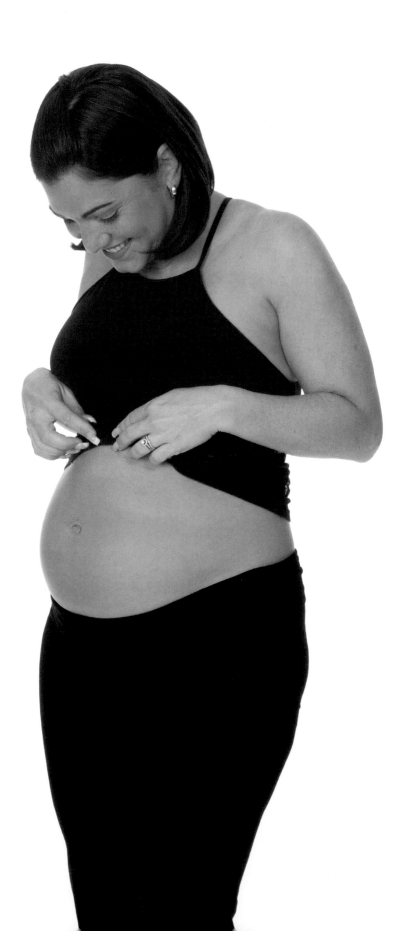

weight, well, it is what it is (and it'll change rapidly). Aim to complete each exercise in about forty-five to sixty seconds before moving on to the next one. If you find that your baby doesn't offer enough resistance, consider using hand weights instead. And if your baby is too heavy for certain moves, put him down in a safe spot and complete the set using light hand weights or no added resistance.

• Watch your baby. If your baby is not yet holding her head up with ease, double-check that your little one's head and neck are fully supported throughout each exercise.

• Check your own body mechanics when exercising with your baby. It's common to sacrifice your own good form in order to hold your baby more securely, especially if an exercise feels quite taxing for you. Avoid pushing your belly out to support your baby or bending your wrists forward or back to hold him close to you. If your form is faltering because you're worried about your baby's comfort and safety, place your baby on a comfy spot on the floor or in a baby seat. Continue the exercise without resistance or pick up a hand weight instead. Try to incorporate your baby into the exercise in a week or so when you feel stronger. *Note: For safety reasons, avoid standing directly above or to the side of your baby when you're using hand weights.*

• Begin every exercise in neutral posture, meaning your body position is well balanced and at its strongest point for safe, effective movement. (See chapter 2, pages 10 to 13, for step-by-step instructions on how to get into a neutral position.)

• When exercising at home, make sure the temperature in your living room or wherever you're working out is comfortable for your baby. You'll start to feel quite toasty as your body heats up from the exercise; however, turning the thermostat down might be more pleasant for you than for your baby.

• Wear supportive shoes that fit your feet as they are now, as opposed to ones that you wore before you were pregnant. The reason: It's common for women's feet to get a bit wider during pregnancy and then stay that way. Don't let ill-fitting footwear interfere with your exercise enjoyment. The same goes for your bra—wear one that's supportive and that fits your current breast size. Digging out the bras you exercised in before you were expecting probably won't work. Overall, dress in comfortable clothes that are meant for exercise. If you're between outfits, a common problem as your body morphs from its pregnancy shape into various postpartum shapes, consider treating yourself to an inexpensive fitness outfit. You can get reasonably priced items at stores like Old Navy or the Gap when you want something new but don't want to break the bank on gear that won't fit in a few months anyway.

• Finally, a few pieces of advice about scheduling exercise: On Sundays, plan your workouts for the week ahead, selecting times when your baby is most likely to be in an agreeable mood—that is, fed, changed, and alert. Be flexible; plan on one or two backup times, just in case. Many of my Baby Boot Camp clients say mornings, between 9 a.m. and noon, work best on most days. However, every baby's different, so experiment with what works in your household. Also, keep in mind that the timing of your baby's best moods will

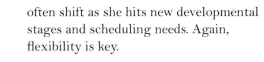

often shift as she hits new developmental stages and scheduling needs. Again, flexibility is key.

The postpartum period may feel a little topsy-turvy to you right now. But it's also a very precious time that gives you a special chance to create lasting healthy habits for you and the ones you love. Your baby will pick up on your lifestyle choices, even at an early age. Showing her that being active is a natural part of everyday life will help her develop important health-enhancing habits of her own.

CHECKLIST FOR GETTING STARTED

Right before you work out, go through the following checklist to ensure the best experience possible for you and your little one. For example, you are more likely to make it through a nine-minute routine one or more times if your baby's belly is full and his diaper is dry and clean. If you're breast-feeding, you'll feel more comfortable doing certain exercises with breasts that aren't too milk-engorged—another good reason to feed baby beforehand.

Make sure:
• Baby's been fed
• Baby's been changed

• Comfort items are within arm's reach (e.g., blanket, burp pad, pacifier, favorite toy)
• Thermostat is set for baby's comfort (indoor workouts)

Remember to bring:
• Toys to occupy baby: activity toys for older babies; soft book or mobile for younger ones
• Snacks, bottle, cup for older babies
• Towel, mat, water bottle for you
• Diapers, wipes, sunscreen, sun hats for you and baby (outdoor workouts)

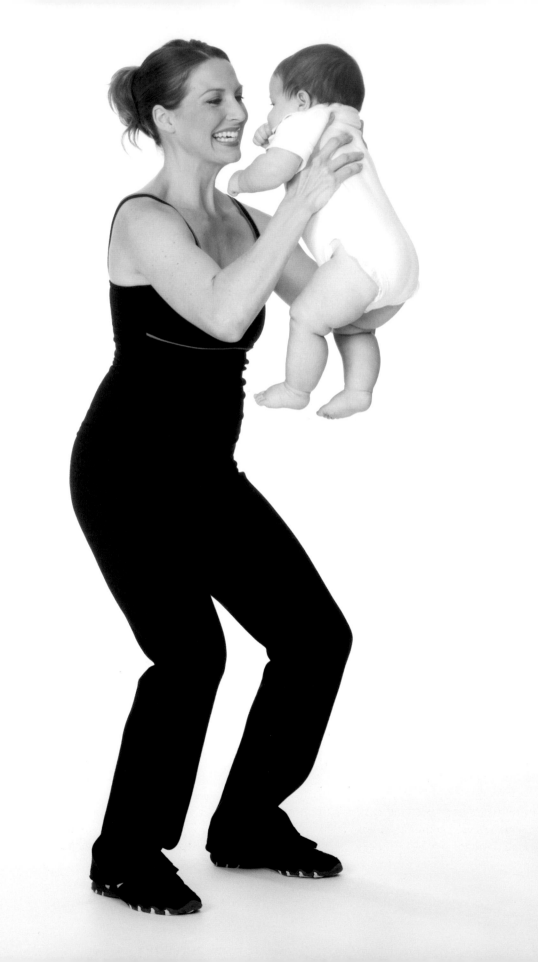

CHAPTER 2

Back-Saving, Tension-Busting Strategies for New Moms

For forty weeks, your body endured incredible transformation to grow a new life. Early on, your waist seemed to all but disappear. Soon, your belly began to protrude, and, before long, your center of gravity was shifting forward. By your third trimester, your pelvis had tipped forward, too, and your ribs had migrated upward to make room for your little one. No doubt about it, over those nine months, your posture changed. And, as you might guess, that change doesn't just reverse itself once your baby is born. In fact, many of the demands you face in these postpartum months can make matters worse!

Just think about a typical day with your newborn. You probably spend most of your time wearing or holding him. When you wear your baby in a front carrier or sling, the baby's weight, your weak postpregnancy back and abs, and your tight chest muscles all make it more likely that you'll end up with shoulders and an upper back that round forward. When you get in the habit of standing or sitting like that, your abs tend to stick out even more, which just makes you appear pregnant all over again!

And then there's how you hold your baby in your arms. It's very common for parents to raise one shoulder while cuddling baby. It sounds innocuous enough, but doing it all the time engages muscles on just one side of the back, neck, and shoulders, which makes them not only uncomfortably tight but also out of balance with other muscles in your upper body. When your baby becomes old enough to hold her head up, you might carry her on one hip, which creates yet another imbalance all the way up and down your body. Even basic activities such as breast-feeding or bottle-feeding, burping baby, carrying a car seat, and stooping over a crib contribute to the postural imbalances you'd rather be counteracting now that your pregnancy's over. Remember from the discussion in chapter 1 that muscle imbalances make injury more likely. What's more, they prevent you from looking and feeling your best.

Now the good news: This chapter will help you improve how your posture looks so you appear leaner, feel less muscular tension, and, most importantly, stave off injury caused by posture-related muscle imbalances. In the exercise chapters to come, you'll learn how to strengthen key muscles that naturally help you move and hold yourself with better posture.

To begin, I invite you to take a look at the difference between neutral posture and typical postpregnancy alignment.

Comparing the two will help you see what it means to establish good body mechanics—whether you gave birth just a few weeks ago or you're well into the postpregnancy months.

What Neutral Posture Is and Why You Need It

The two photos on page 11 shed light on just how much pregnancy affects posture. See how in the photo on the left, my ears, shoulders, hips, knees, and ankles are all in line? Notice, also, how the spine follows a subtle and natural curvature. There's a tiny arch in the lower back, the upper back rounds out slightly, then the spine curves in just a bit again at the neck. The pelvis is positioned so that the two hip bones and the pubic bone face directly forward.

This is an example of *neutral posture*, where muscle and postural imbalances are minimized. In neutral, your body is optimally positioned for safe and efficient movement. (I teach you the simple steps for getting yourself into neutral posture in the sidebar on page 12.)

Your posture probably looked something like the model shown in the photo on the left before you got pregnant. I say "something like" because, pregnancy aside, most people have trouble sticking to good posture. A sedentary lifestyle, hours sitting at a computer, and long commutes are just a few of the factors that wreak havoc on posture—pregnancy or no pregnancy. So now's the perfect opportunity to come out of your recent pregnancy looking better than ever!

Does the pose in the photo on the right look familiar? This is the typical stance for someone who's at about 6 weeks postpartum, but can stick with you for years. Here's how you get that way: As your belly grows, your pelvis begins to naturally tilt forward. Once your pelvis tips out of neutral, the spine follows. The lower spine gets pulled forward, creating a larger-than-normal arch in the lower back. When the lower back dips inward like that, the upper back rounds more, which, in turn, causes your head to jut forward.

Looking in the mirror, you've probably noticed how pregnancy has changed the way you stand (and sit). You may also be aware of how this postural shift feels. Perhaps some body parts are especially tight while others seem soft and weak. The imbalances of postpregnancy posture tend to tighten muscles in the

• neck (at the back)
• front of the shoulders
• chest
• lower back
• front of the hips (hip flexors)

Meanwhile, other muscles weaken and may get too stretched-out. These include muscles in the

• neck (at the front)
• back of your shoulders
• upper back
• abs
• butt
• hamstrings

Apart from making you feel better, developing proper posture helps you move in the most efficient way possible. Starting any exercise or everyday activity in a neutral position allows you to zone in on the right muscles, so you work what you want to work and don't unintentionally make muscle imbalances worse, instead of better. For example, if you do standing biceps curls while your pelvis is tilted forward (not

Left: Neutral posture.

Right: A typical stance for someone who is about 16 weeks postpartum.

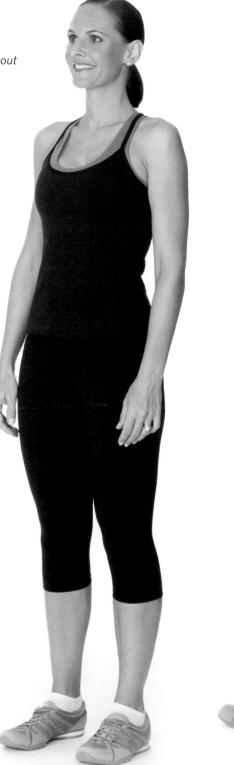
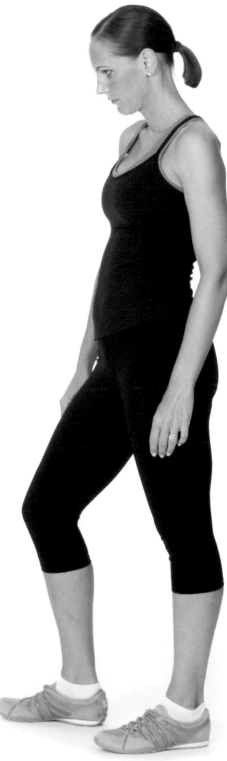

On Neutral Ground

Good posture makes you look good, and it prevents aches and pains because proper body alignment–or what I'm calling neutral posture–places the least stress on your muscles and joints. To practice a neutral stance, try the following posture check. I teach it in all my Baby Boot Camp classes.

• Begin with your feet hip-width apart and knees "soft" (i.e., your legs are straight but your knees aren't locked).

• Tilt your pelvis forward and backward. First create a large arch in the lower back, then make your lower back as flat as you can. Settle your pelvis between these two extremes so there's only a slight curve in your lower back. Your tailbone should point toward the floor and your hip bones should face directly forward.

• Place your palms on the front of your pelvis (where your hip bones are) and tighten your abs by gently drawing your belly button toward your spine. (See the "Tummy Tuck" move in chapter 3, page 22, and the photo.)

• Round your upper back, then do the opposite by squeezing your shoulder blades together. Position your shoulder blades between these two extremes.

• Gently lower your shoulder blades toward the floor.

• Pull your chin back so your ears line up over your shoulders. Lengthen the top of your head toward the ceiling, creating space between your ears and your shoulders.

Practicing the "Tummy Tuck."

neutral), you're more likely to initiate the movement using your lower back when what you really want is to engage your abs as you work your arms. The same concept applies to lifting your baby, a diaper bag, a stroller, a car seat, and any other hefty baby gear.

Prepping Your Posture for Day-to-Day Activities with Baby

There's no sense in getting your posture right for exercise only to forget all about it in everyday life! Setting up and maintaining good posture is just as important for your day-to-day activities. Here are tips for prepping your posture for some of your biggest demands as a new mom.

Feeding Baby

Whether you breast-feed, bottle-feed or do a combination, you may be prone to hunching over your baby as he enjoys a meal. Perhaps you've been unconsciously sacrificing your posture to ensure that your baby is properly positioned at the breast. Or maybe your upper body and back simply aren't well-supported. Either way, figuring out the right posture for this day-and-night duty will go a long way toward cutting out backaches and doing away with that typical postpregnancy slouch.

• Your first step is to assemble the right upper-body and back support so when you sit down for a feed, your posture-saving props are already there for you. Create a nursing "station" for yourself and your baby that includes a firm nursing pillow and a lumbar-support cushion.

• Next, look at your feet. Do they reach the floor comfortably when your back is fully supported? If not, use a low footstool. Your knees should be aligned with your hips, your thighs parallel to the floor.

Wearing Baby

Wearing your baby in a sling or front carrier may contribute to a rounded upper back and shoulders that slump forward. In later chapters, we'll get to exercises that strengthen the muscles in your upper body and torso so this posture isn't such a problem. But there's also something you can do sooner: The next time you wear your baby, follow the two posture-enhancing steps below. (**Hint:** These are some of the steps you take to get neutral posture.)

• Straighten your back and tighten your abs by contracting your belly button toward your spine without squeezing your butt muscles.

The correct posture for feeding your baby.

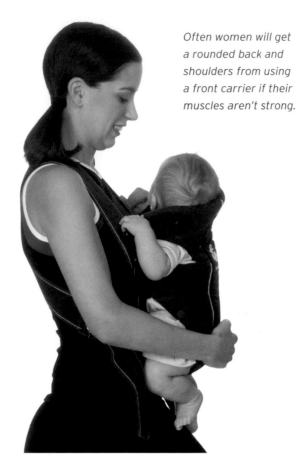

Often women will get a rounded back and shoulders from using a front carrier if their muscles aren't strong.

- Make a point of holding your baby on the side you favor the least often for at least twenty seconds at a time, three times a day.

- Neutral posture can apply to your wrists, too. Avoid achy wrists or aggravating carpal tunnel syndrome (a common occurrence in expecting women) by ensuring that your wrists aren't bent forward or backward when they don't need to be. For example, hold your baby so your wrists are straight. The same advice goes for bottle-feeding.

- To prevent raising one shoulder when cuddling baby, get in the habit of drawing both your shoulders away from your ears right after you pick up your baby.

- If you are holding your baby with, say, just your right arm, reach your left arm across your body to support your right arm. This lets you relax your right wrist a bit, which helps take the pressure off that joint.

- Draw your shoulder blades down toward your hips as far as they can go. Lift your chest and squeeze your shoulder blades toward each other. Release these extreme positions about halfway until your upper back feels strong but not tense.

Lifting and Holding Baby

You've probably noticed that you favor lifting and holding your baby with one arm over the other. It's only natural. However, this habit increases the possibility of muscle imbalances and common postpregnancy repetitive-strain injuries, such as carpal tunnel syndrome. To help balance work and rest time between your dominant and nondominant shoulder, arm, hand, and wrist, try these suggestions:

A better way of lifting and holding your baby.

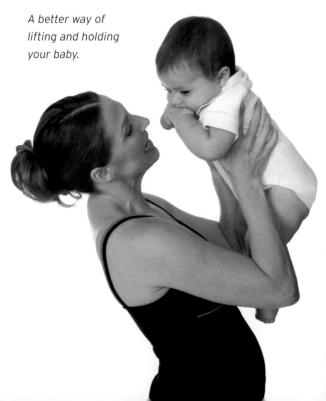

Carrying the Car Seat

Lugging around a bulky car seat is a real pain in the neck . . . and the back . . . and the shoulders. There doesn't seem to be any way to get it right, either. If you hold the car seat's handle, your wrist can easily bend into an awkward position. You might try to avoid that problem by looping the handle over your forearm. But then you risk cutting off circulation and bruising your forearm. As if that weren't enough, there's also the common habit of stabilizing the car seat on one hip. This does lessen stress on the joints in the arms, but it puts your pelvis off-kilter. From there, you have no chance at holding neutral posture. The fix? Try my tips below:

• First, consider that a car seat is not meant to be a baby carrier.

• With the above point in mind, carry the car seat without baby in it whenever possible to create a slightly lighter load. If you can, safely remove baby from her car seat and snuggle her into her stroller instead of taking the seat and the baby out of the car all at once.

• If the car seat affixes on the stroller or you don't have your stroller with you, the above system might not work for you. In that case, consider cuddling your baby into a front carrier to save your body from carting her in the car seat. Your baby prefers to travel as close to you as possible anyway.

Stroller-Walking

I encourage you to go stroller-walking whenever you can. It's an easy, baby-friendly way to squeeze exercise into your day. Still, how you push the stroller and grip the handle can promote bad posture. Remember the following acronym for proper stroller-pushing form: W.A.S.H.

W = Wrists neutral. Place your hands on the push bar with your wrists in neutral alignment—that is, you shouldn't be bending the wrists forward or backward.

A = Abs in. When facing forward with the stroller in front of you, imagine pulling your belly button away from the stroller and toward your spine.

S = Shoulders down. Take a deep breath and relax your shoulders. Think about creating space between your ears and your shoulders.

H = Hips forward. Keep the stroller—and, therefore, your baby—close to your hips so you're less prone to slouching forward and using your back to gain leverage when walking up an incline or hill.

With these posture primers, you can lay the foundation for getting back in shape, efficiently and safely. So strike a neutral stance, and start the next section: your life as a fit mom!

Remember to push your stroller using the correct form.

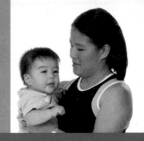

PART 2

Baby Boot Camp Exercises

CHAPTER 3

Your Baby Is Six to Twelve Weeks Old

As a mom with a very young infant, you're probably adjusting to the first dizzying weeks of childbirth recovery, new parenthood, and/or caring for a newborn (and perhaps other kids, too). Right now, squeezing in an unwavering workout schedule simply isn't realistic, and there's no reason to feel guilty about it. So there you have it. No guilt, please!

That's not to say you should let yourself entirely off the hook (after all, you're reading this book, which shows you're serious about getting back in shape). I encourage you to follow the fitness guidelines in this chapter as closely as you can. Exercising in the early postpartum stage will help you feel better and bounce back faster. However, it's OK to be flexible. If you manage to work in three workouts one week and only one workout the next week, so be it. Just regard each new day as another chance to get moving.

And don't forget that the routine in this chapter can help with a common imperative for new moms: calming a fussy baby. You might be pleasantly surprised by your baby's positive reaction to the rhythmic motion of the squats on page 26 or how well he settles when you cuddle him into your chest to do the bridge exercise on page 31.

By now, you're probably getting a clear picture of how your baby will factor into the Baby Boot Camp fitness plan. Let's take a look at what he might be up to in this six- to twelve-week phase, and how these developments play into the exercises you'll find on the following pages.

What's Happening, Baby?

At this early stage, your baby is unable to hold his head up (and he won't be able to for a few months more). So make sure his tiny head is well-supported during each exercise.

It's safest to put your baby on his back when he sleeps, but he also needs time on his tummy when he's awake to help strengthen his neck muscles enough to eventually hold his head up. If you elect not to hold or wear your baby during some exercises, consider giving him "tummy time" on a safe, comfy spot on the floor.

You might notice your baby is starting to smile in a social way now. To encourage social and emotional interaction and heart-melting smiles, look your baby in the face, smile, coo, and be expressive as you work out. The more you make exercise time enjoyable for both of you, the more motivated you'll be to actually do it.

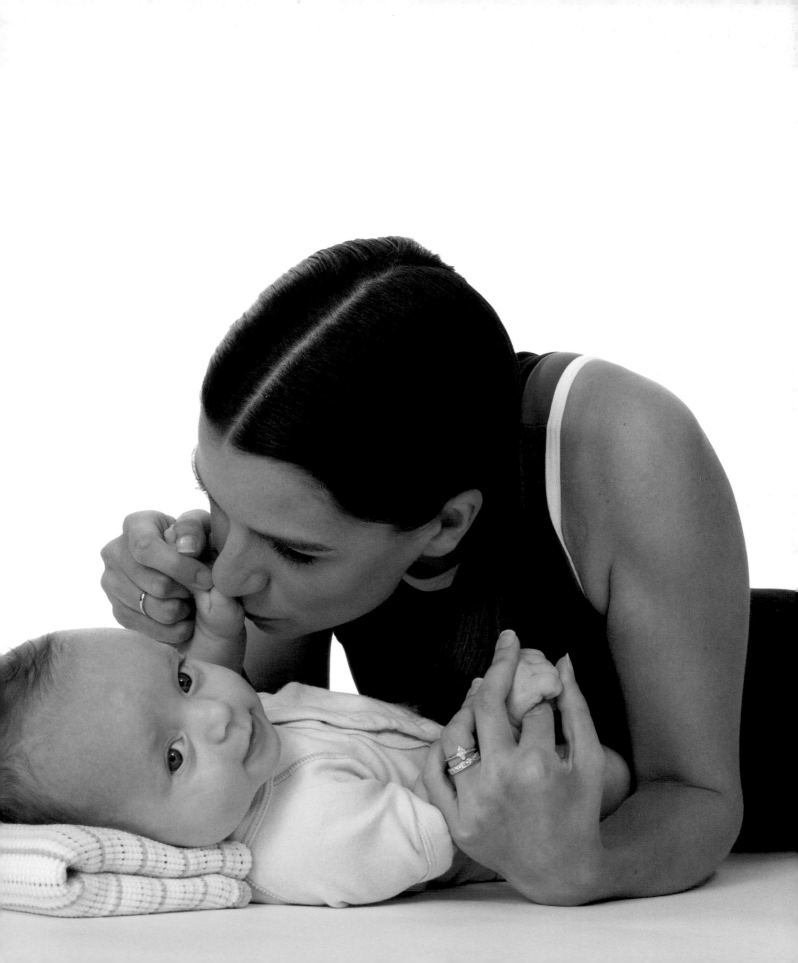

Finally, as the weeks go by, you might observe that your baby starts to sleep less during the day. Plan your workouts accordingly, depending on whether you prefer to work out with your baby (as shown on the following pages) or solo (or even a bit of both). If you want the added incentive of seeing how much more weight you are able to lift over time (a sign that you and your baby are getting stronger), fill in your baby's weight at right.

How to Get Started

Postchildbirth exercise should progress gradually, according to the American College of Obstetricians and Gynecologists (ACOG). In consideration of this recommendation, the chapter you're reading offers one nine-minute strength routine you can do for the next six weeks or so (at about twelve weeks postpartum, it'll be time to flip over to chapter 4). I've designed only one routine for this postpartum phase because you'll have enough going on in these six weeks as it is. Mastering the first nine exercises and "The Basic Three" (more on these in a minute) will be plenty.

In keeping with industry standards (including those at Baby Boot Camp), I encourage you to wait until six weeks after delivery to begin this workout (if you've had a cesarean section, you may need to wait until eight weeks, depending on how your recovery is progressing).

If you're reading this chapter before you've hit the six-week postnatal milestone, I encourage you to do just "The Basic Three" exercises described on pages 22 and 23. "The Basic Three" are a trio of essential exercises for preventing injury, getting your abs back in shape (and making sure they lie flat), and controlling urinary leakage. The best part about "The Basic Three" is that you can do them as you nurse or bottle-feed,

WHAT YOU'RE LIFTING THESE DAYS: YOUR BABY'S WEIGHT

WEEK	WEIGHT	DATE
6		
7		
8		
9		
10		
11		
12		

during diaper changes or while you go about any number of baby-related duties. So you don't have to carve out extra time in your day to start seeing positive results from "The Basic Three."

What about Diastasis Recti?

You might notice that you have *diastasis recti*, which is a gap between the two halves of the muscle along the front and middle of your abdomen. It's not uncommon for some women to develop this condition during pregnancy or even as a result of the pushing phase during childbirth—but it shouldn't be ignored now that you've had your baby. To test if you have it, lie faceup—legs bent, feet flat on the floor—and do an abdominal crunch, bringing your head and shoulders off the floor. If you have diastasis recti, you'll feel a two- to three-inch (5–7.5cm) ridge, bulge, or separation about one to two inches (2.5–5cm) above or below your belly button.

If you find that you have this condition, here's what to do: Perform the Tummy Tuck exercise as directed in this chapter (do it frequently throughout your day). It's important to build a strong foundation of strength and stability in your deep abs so your outer abs can properly recover.

In these early postpartum months, you may also need to steer clear of or modify movements like the ab crunch (except when testing for this condition). All the exercises I've included in chapters 3 and 4 are safe for you to do if you have diastasis recti.

EXERCISE GUIDELINES FOR THIS CHAPTER

Read the steps below for what to expect from the workout in this chapter.

• Get warmed up with the moves described on pages 22 and 23.

• After your warm-up, aim to do each strength exercise for about forty-five to sixty seconds.

• Follow this chapter's nine-minute routine every other day (or as close to that schedule as possible from week to week). This works out to be three to four times a week.

• If you're able to do the routine in this chapter at least three times a week for two weeks in a row, try running through the routine two times back to back to boost intensity (if you have the energy and baby agrees to an extended workout, of course).

• Commit to doing each move in "The Basic Three" (pages 22 and 23) at least three times a day. This is in addition to your nine-minute strength routine.

• See the cardio workout, which you can do outside, with your baby in her stroller, at the end of this chapter.

• You'll find stretching exercises specifically for the postpartum body in chapter 7. Do these moves after every strength and cardio workout or whenever you can fit in one or more stretches throughout the day.

The Basic Three

Do each of the following three exercises at least three times a day when you have a calm, quiet moment to yourself (yeah, right!) or while carrying out baby-related tasks like feedings, diapers changes, and the like.

Combined, these moves help:
• make your abs feel stronger and lie flatter
• prevent or control incontinence
• improve your posture and make you look better
• cut down on backaches and your overall risk of injury

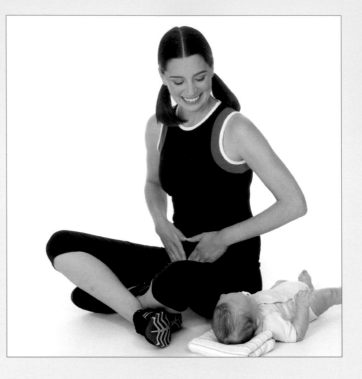

1. Tummy Tuck

Works: the deep abdominal muscle, called the transverse abdominis

Stand, lie faceup, or sit in a chair or on the floor. Place your palms on your lower abdominal muscles with your thumbs touching and your index (pointer) fingers touching to form a triangle shape. Take a deep breath in and relax your abs. As you breathe out, tighten and flatten your abs, as if drawing your belly button toward your spine. You should feel your lower abs gently pull away from your hands. Repeat this sequence nine times.

2. Kegels*

Works: the pelvic floor

These are the muscles you'd use to stop the flow of urine. (*Note:* Kegels do not mean routinely stopping the flow of urine. Try it one time just to get a feel for how to contract your pelvic floor, which gets stretched and weakened after pregnancy and a vaginal delivery.)

Basic Kegels
Begin in a standing, lying, or sitting position. Squeeze the pelvic floor muscles upward. Hold for five seconds, breathing normally. Over time, increase how long you hold the Kegel. Once you feel comfortable doing the Basic Kegel described above, alternate it with the following variations.

Elevator Kegels
Imagine that the muscles of your vagina are a building. The base of your pelvic floor is the lobby and your belly button is the top floor. Slowly raise the "elevator" floor by floor, lifting and tightening the pelvic-floor muscles. At the top floor (belly button), hold for one to two seconds, then slowly lower the elevator, relaxing the pelvic floor from top to bottom.

Sustained Kegels
Contract the pelvic floor for ten seconds and then relax it, repeating ten times. If you have trouble holding the contraction for ten seconds at first, work up to it over time.

Progressive Kegels
Squeeze the pelvic floor for five seconds, then squeeze a little harder, holding for another five seconds. Release and repeat two more times.

*Kegels might not be right for every woman who's recently given birth. If you already feel pain in the pelvic or perineal region, Kegels may make this discomfort worse. Consult your physician, midwife, or a pelvic-pain specialist if Kegels cause or worsen pain or discomfort.

3. Shoulder Blade Squeezes

Works: the muscles in the middle of your back that help you stand/sit with good posture and prevent your shoulders from rounding forward

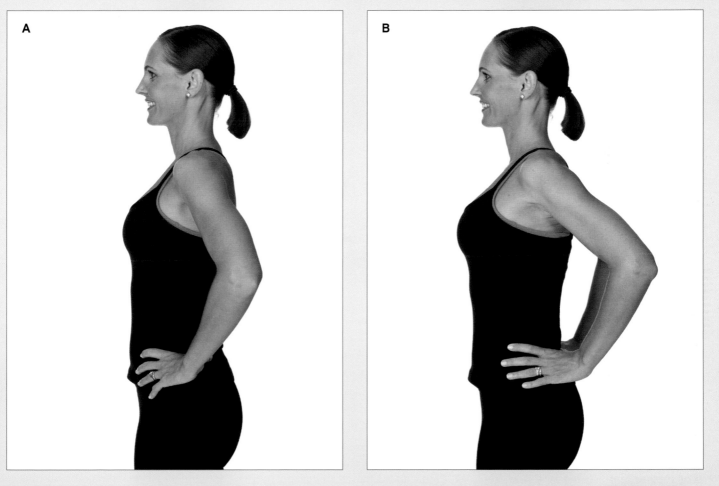

A. Stand or sit with your shoulders relaxed and hands on hips.

B. In a standing or sitting position, tighten your abs (see Tummy Tuck move on opposite page). Squeeze your shoulder blades toward each other and toward your spine without allowing your shoulders to rise. Visualize holding a pencil between your shoulder blades. Isolate this movement in your back, keeping your hands on your hips. Hold this position for three seconds. Relax and repeat.

Marches with Half-Squats

Do it for: three minutes total

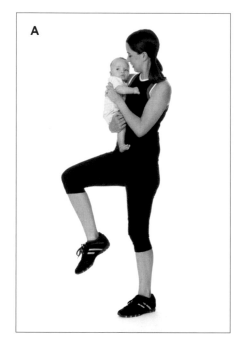

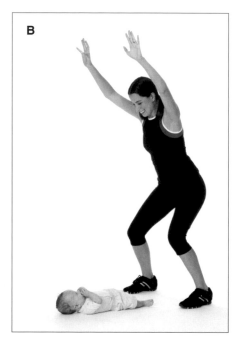

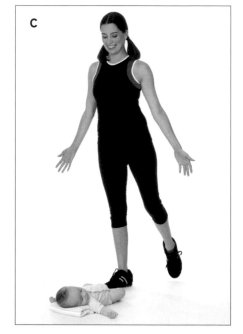

A. Minute 1:
Preparing for Marches with Half-Squats.

1. Hold your baby in your arms or settle her on the floor and step far enough away from her so you can safely and comfortably move on the spot. Make sure she can see you!

2. March in place, pumping your arms at your sides for thirty seconds. If you're wearing your baby, use one or both arms to support her head and to shield her body from any jarring movements.

3. Place your hands on your hips, with your feet hip-width apart. Do half-squats with your buttocks pushing behind you as if you were just starting to sit down in a chair. Continue for thirty seconds.

B. Minute 2:
Half-squats with arm movements.

1. Keep doing the half-squats but this time add the arm movements shown in the photo above: Raise your arms overhead, reaching toward the ceiling every time you squat. Repeat for thirty seconds.

2. Return to the march on the spot, pumping your arms at your sides for thirty seconds.

C. Minute 3:
Half-squats with a leg lift.

1. Go back to the half-squats. This time, lift your leg behind your body after each half-squat, as shown in the photo above. As you lift your leg behind your body, stretch your arms to the sides and squeeze your shoulder blades, palms forward. Keep your shoulders relaxed and your hands just below shoulder height. Repeat for thirty seconds.

2. March on the spot for the final thirty seconds.

Reach & Pull

Works: upper and midback

Making It Work with Baby: Wear your baby in a front carrier or sling, or place your baby on the floor in front of you (with her feet closest to you) so she can gaze up at your face.

C-Section Considerations: Reduce the amount you round forward at the spine if it makes your incision feel uncomfortable.

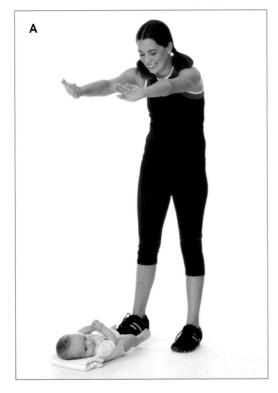

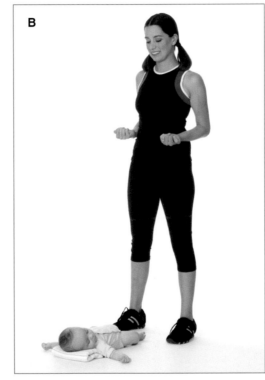

TRAINER TIP

Avoid lifting your shoulder blades during this exercise. Try a few reps in front of the mirror to make sure that your shoulders stay down.

A. Stand with feet hip-width apart, reaching your arms in front of your body. Your arms should be parallel to the floor and your hands slightly below your shoulders. Reach your arms away from your body a bit more as you round through your spine.

B. Straighten your spine and bend your elbows, pulling your arms toward your body in a rowing motion as you squeeze your shoulder blades toward each other; hold for three counts. Return to starting position and repeat.

Sit-Down Squats

Works: thighs, buttocks

Making It Work with Baby: Hold your baby close to your chest, supporting his head with your hand, or wear him in a front carrier or sling with your arms reaching in front of you.

C-Section Considerations: If you feel discomfort at the incision site when you squat because of how your baby is positioned in a sling or front carrier, try shifting the baby's position slightly. If the discomfort persists, shorten your range of motion so you aren't squatting low enough to touch the chair behind you.

TRAINER TIP

Focus on sitting down into the squat motion. Your knees should not push past your toes.

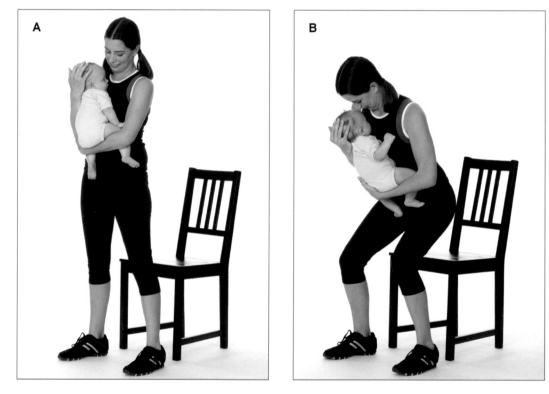

A. Stand in front of a sturdy chair with your feet hip-width apart, knees facing forward.

B. Bend your knees, sitting back as if you were going to sit in the chair behind you.

Lightly touch your bottom to the chair before straightening your legs to return to a standing position. Repeat this movement.

Arm Circles

Works: shoulders

Making It Work with Baby: Wear your baby in a front carrier or sling. If she's facing forward, do this exercise in front of the mirror so she can see you. Or place your baby on the floor in front of you (with her feet closest to you) so she can watch you.

C-Section Considerations: Keep your deep ab muscles engaged throughout this exercise to help facilitate the healing of your lower abdominals and speed your recovery time.

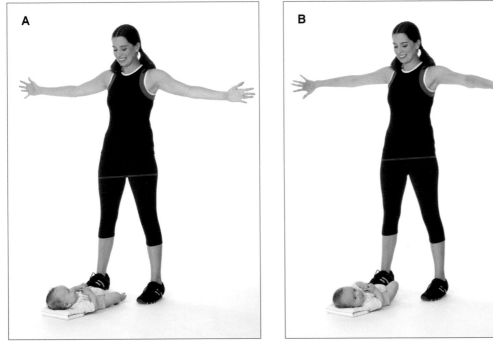

🌸 **TRAINER TIP**
Keep your abs tight, stand up straight, and squeeze your shoulder blades slightly together.

A. Stand with your feet hip-width apart and your arms horizontal to the floor and extended at your sides, hands just below shoulder height. Begin with your palms facing forward, thumbs up. Make little circular motions in the air with your arms for twenty seconds.

B. Rotate your palms upward, thumbs pointing back, and make little circular motions for another twenty seconds before rotating your palms downward, thumbs pointing forward, making little arms circles for a final twenty seconds. Repeat the sequence.

Supermom

Works: low back, back of legs, buttocks

Making It Work with Baby: Place baby on the floor in front of you, reaching for his hands.

C-Section Considerations: If lying facedown on your incision just doesn't feel right, skip this move and do an extra set of the Four-Point Kneeling exercise instead (see opposite page).

✿ TRAINER TIP

Unless you're looking up to see how your baby is doing, keep your neck neutral so you're facing the floor throughout this exercise. Be careful to not hyperextend your spine by lifting too high.

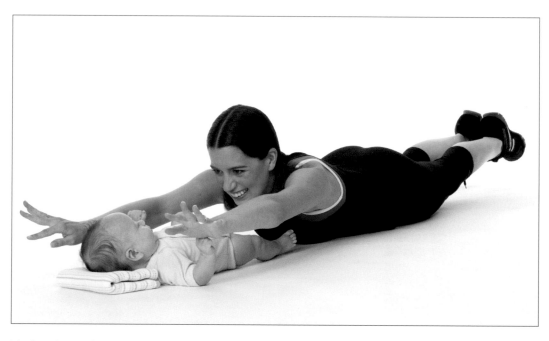

Lie facedown with your arms extended over your head, palms facing inward, and your legs straight, toes pointed. Activate your abs by tightening your entire abdominal area as if you were wearing snug-fitting jeans.

Lift both arms about six to eight inches (15–20.5cm) off the floor. Keeping your arms hovering in the air, lift both legs about six to eight inches (15–20.5cm) off the floor.

Slowly lower arms and legs to the floor. Repeat.

Four-Point Kneeling*

Works: abs, back, buttocks

Making It Work with Baby: Place your baby on her back with your hands on either side of her body so she can gaze directly up into your face.

C-Section Considerations: Make your leg lifts smaller if you feel a slight pulling sensation around your incision.

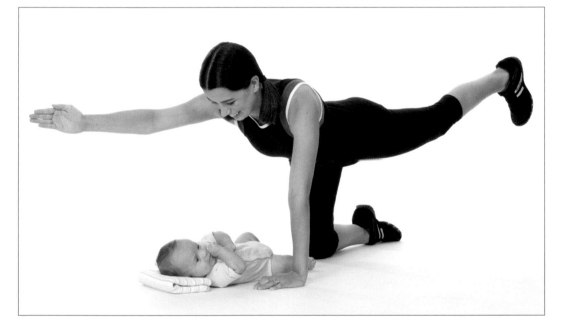

🌸 TRAINER TIP
Keep your back straight and your abs tight. If you're wobbling too much to hold good form, practice lifting the arm and the leg one at a time.

Kneel on all fours with your hands and knees on the floor. Align your hands under your shoulders and your knees under your hips. Then, with your abs contracted, raise your right arm, palm facing inward, and your left leg, foot flexed, until both are parallel to the floor. Hold for three seconds, as shown. Return to the starting position and repeat with left arm and right leg. Alternate sides.

Modification for wrist pain or discomfort with Four-Point Kneeling and Kiss-Your-Baby Push-ups: Instead of completing this exercise with flat palms, keep your wrists straight by placing your knuckles on a folded-up towel on the floor.

Kiss-Your-Baby Push-ups*

Works: abs, chest, shoulders, arms

Making It Work with Baby: Place your baby faceup on the floor between your hands, aligning her face under yours. Every time you lower yourself toward the floor, give her a big kiss on the cheek.

C-Section Considerations: If you feel pulling or other discomfort around the incision, keep your hips bent as you lower your chest toward the floor.

TRAINER TIP

Not ready to get low enough for kisses? Try this modified push-up instead: Bend your arms to about forty-five degrees and look into your baby's eyes. Smile.

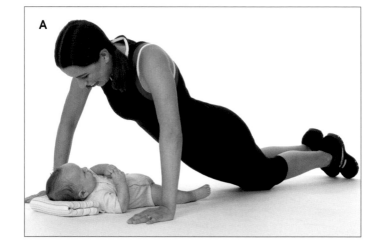

A. Kneel on all fours with your hands and knees on the floor. Place your hands a little wider than shoulder-width apart.

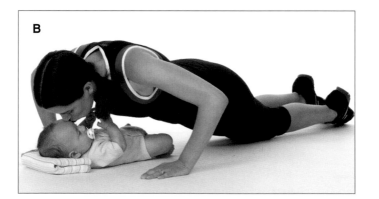

B. Contract your abs and straighten your hips. Slowly bend your arms to about ninety degrees, bringing your chest toward the floor and keeping your back and neck straight and your abs tight, as shown. Then straighten your arms to return to the starting position. Repeat.

Modification for wrist pain or discomfort with Four-Point Kneeling and Kiss-Your-Baby Push-ups: Instead of completing this exercise with flat palms, keep your wrists straight by placing your knuckles on a folded-up towel on the floor.

Baby Bridges

Works: low back, backs of thighs, buttocks

Making It Work with Baby: Snuggle your newborn close to your chest, making sure to support his head and shoulders with your hands.

C-Section Considerations: Be careful not to push your pelvis too high in the air, which might make the incision feel uncomfortable, as if it's being stretched. Controlling the position of your pelvis will also help prevent your lower back from overarching.

A. Lie faceup with your legs bent and the soles of your feet flat on the floor. Place your heels about twelve inches (30.5cm) from your buttocks.

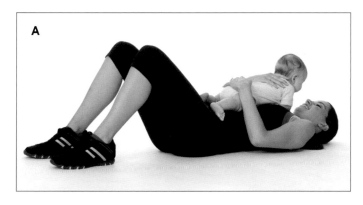

TRAINER TIP

Squeeze your butt muscles to make the most out of this bridge exercise. Doing so helps create a firm butt and prevents your low spine from dipping toward the floor and your pelvis from tilting side to side.

B. Slowly raise your hips off the floor, squeezing your butt muscles and keeping your spine straight (not curving in or out). Your feet, shoulder blades, and head should remain on the floor. Hold this bridge position for three seconds before lowering your hips back to the floor. Repeat.

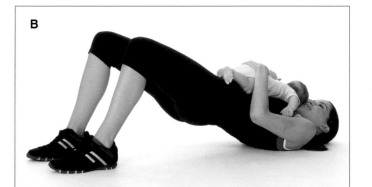

Heel Slides

Works: abs

Making It Work with Baby: Hold your baby against your chest. Support her head with your hands.

C-Section Considerations: If the area around your incision feels strained or as if it's pulling during this exercise, shorten your range of motion so you aren't straightening your leg all the way.

TRAINER TIP

Avoid allowing your low spine to arch upward and away from the floor. Contract your abs to keep your low back close to the floor.

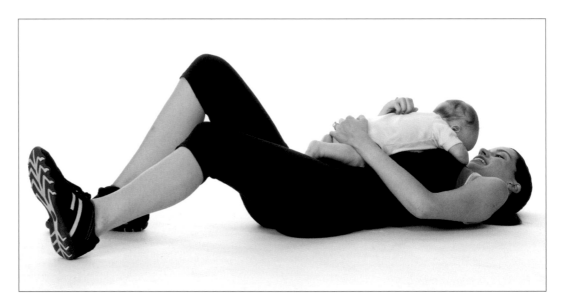

Lie on your back with your knees bent and your feet flat on the floor. Tighten your abs and slowly straighten your right leg, sliding your right foot away from your body.

Bring your right foot back to the starting position. Keeping your abs tight, straighten your left leg, sliding the left foot away from the body. Return to the starting position and repeat, alternating sides.

Tummy Tuck & Kegel Combo

Works: abs, pelvic floor muscles

Making It Work with Baby: Place baby on the floor beside you. You'll need your hands free so you can place them on your lower abs (this will help you learn how to properly contract your abs).

C-Section Considerations: If touching your abs near the incision feels uncomfortable, adjust your hand placement.

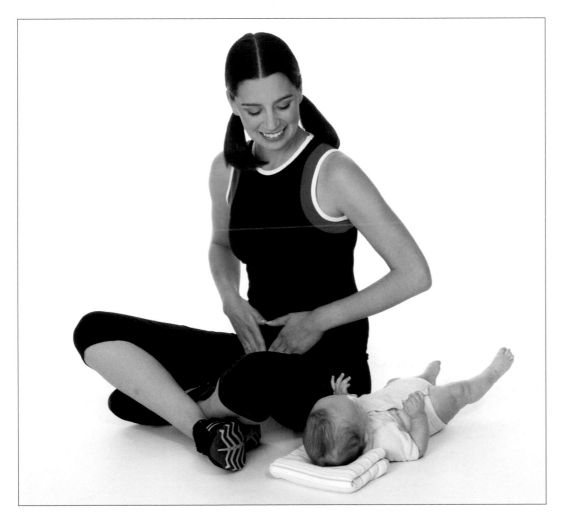

🌸 TRAINER TIP
Don't hold your breath! Breathe normally as you maintain this powerful combo contraction.

Lie faceup or sit on the floor, placing both palms between your two hip bones on your lower abdominals. Take a deep breath in and relax your abs. As you breathe out, tighten and flatten your abs, drawing your belly button toward your spine. You should feel your lower abs gently pull away from your hands. Without letting go of the ab contraction, squeeze the pelvic floor muscles upward. Hold for five to ten seconds; relax and repeat the sequence.

29-Minute Cardio Workout

Do this cardio workout three times a week with your baby in a stroller or a front carrier. Check that you are at the right intensity with the
• "talk test" (you should be able to comfortably speak to your baby without gasping for air)
• Rating of Perceived Exertion (RPE) chart below

Rating of Perceived Exertion (RPE)

Use this chart to gauge how much effort to put into your cardio workouts. You should never be at a 1 or a 10. And you will rarely be at a 2 or a 9, either. Aim to work out between an RPE of 3 and 8. The chart below shows you what each level should feel like.

1. no effort
2. minimal, light effort
3. very easy, feels comfortable
4. light to moderate effort
5. moderate to strong effort; you become aware of your breathing
6. strong effort; your breathing is deep and you can't comfortably carry on a conversation
7. very strong effort; you can only talk in short sentences
8. challenging effort; difficult to say more than a few words at a time
9. unable to talk; can only maintain this intensity for very short bouts
10. maxed out, lightheaded, nauseous

What You Need:
• supportive shoes
• water bottle
• your baby in a stroller or front carrier
• a watch that shows time in seconds

Warm-Up

Do it for: five minutes

Walk at a moderate pace, keeping your shoulders back, your spine long (not rounded) and your stroller (if you're using one) close to your hips.

Drill 1:
Thirty/Sixty-Second Intervals

Do it for: 4.5 minutes

Interval A: Walk at a challenging pace for thirty seconds. Your RPE should be 5.

Interval B: Walk for sixty seconds at a slower pace, slowing your breathing and lengthening your steps. Your RPE should be 4.

Alternate Intervals A and B, three times total. Then move on to Drill 2 (see opposite page).

Tip for walking with a stroller: Keep your shoulders back and tighten your abs as you push the stroller (yes, you can and should work your abs even when you're pushing a stroller!).

Tip for walking with a carrier: You might find yourself pushing your belly out as a way to support your baby in the carrier. But you want to train your abs to lie flat, not bulge forward! To correct, make sure the carrier is properly adjusted for your and your baby's size. You may also need to place one hand on your baby for extra support.

Drill 2:
Fifteen/Thirty-Second Intervals

Do it for: six minutes

Interval C: Walk for fifteen seconds at a challenging pace, moving quickly and with slightly longer steps so you raise your heart rate. Your RPE should be 6.

Interval D: Slow down to a moderate pace for thirty seconds to recover from Interval C. Your RPE should be 5.

Alternate Intervals C and D, eight times total.

Tip for walking with a stroller: If you find yourself kicking the stroller when you take long strides, consider using a jogging-style stroller. These models have a wider wheel base in the back so your feet have more room when you step forward. See Appendix B for more on selecting a good exercise stroller.

Tip for walking with a carrier: Strollers usually have one or more built-in sun protectors, but carriers don't. So use sun protection if the weather calls for it: sunscreen and a hat for you, and a wide-brimmed hat and/or a light blanket for your baby.

Repeat Drill 1 (another 4.5 minutes).

Repeat Drill 2 (another six minutes).

Cooldown

Do it for: three minutes

Walk at an easy pace, taking deep breaths. Squeeze your shoulder blades slightly toward each other and hold them like that, so you feel a mild stretch in the front of your shoulders and your chest muscles.

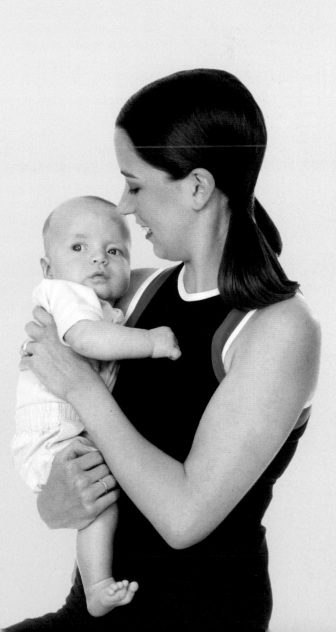

CHAPTER 4

Your Baby Is Three to Five Months Old

I t's official—you've just about made it through your first "trimester" of postpartum life! You're probably feeling almost or completely back to your old self after the delivery. And you might have heard from other parents that it only gets easier from here . . . could the three-month mark be a postpartum panacea of sorts?

Well, perhaps *easier* isn't quite the right word. After all, you'll still face nonstop laundry, interrupted sleep, and dirty diapers. But the good news is, you'll find that parenting an infant gets more manageable as you continue to decipher your baby's cues, understand his budding personality, and fall into some type of a routine. Part of this routine is discovering fun, new ways to bond with your baby while modeling a healthy, fit lifestyle. (At Baby Boot Camp, we think it's never too early to set a good example.)

If you've been diligently doing the previous chapter's exercises, great. If you've let that routine slide a little, fine. Don't beat yourself up about it. But now's the time to start a new chapter—literally—and make serious headway with getting your prebaby body back or getting in even better shape than you were a year ago. One tip: Do your very best to keep up with "The Basic Three"

exercises from chapter 3 (see pages 22 and 23) by continuing to incorporate them into your current activities now and in the coming months.

So let's begin with a look at what your baby might be up to these days, and how her age relates to the exercises you'll be doing for the next three months or so.

What's Happening, Baby?

At about three months, your baby becomes more responsive to her surroundings. She may lift her head while on her tummy and—as her vision improves—show more interest in observing nearby people and objects. She can see details in your face more clearly now, like your lips as you smile. These days, your baby might also enjoy looking over your shoulder when

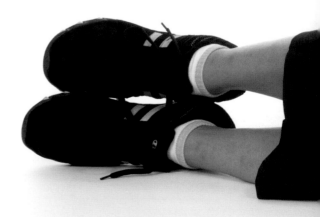

WHAT YOU'RE LIFTING THESE DAYS: YOUR BABY'S WEIGHT		
WEEKS	**WEIGHT**	**DATE**
13-14		
15-16		
17-18		
19-20		
21-23		
24-26		
27-29		

you cuddle her against your chest, as you might do during the Lunge exercise in this chapter. She can track moving objects, such as your hand gestures or a bright, patterned toy dangling from above.

By four months, your baby is moving more. You might notice that when you place your baby on his back while you warm up for exercise or do plié-squats, he'll happily kick his legs and wave his arms around as if he were doing his own workout. He may be able to sit with your support or propped up against pillows. When you sit him on your pelvis during the Bridge exercise in this chapter, he'll get to really gaze at what interests him most—you.

Once your baby is around five months old, he may show the first signs of rolling from his stomach onto his back, or vice versa. He may have already mastered rolling at least one way. Try making common facial expressions at him during the face-to-face exercises in this chapter and see if he imitates you. Your baby has an easier time sitting up now, but you'll still want to support him with your arms and hands during the exercises on these pages.

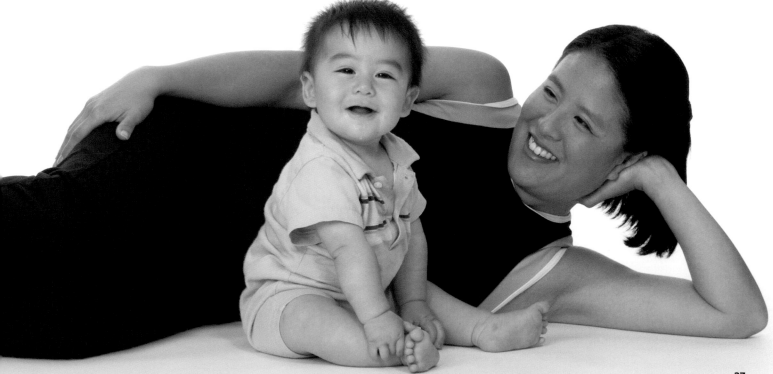

How to Get Started

There are two head-to-toe strength routines in this chapter. Follow the warm-up instructions on the next page; then try Routine 1 for about three weeks. Move on to Routine 2 for the next three weeks (this one you'll do with hand weights so you won't be holding your baby). After that, alternate between the two nine-minute routines in this chapter every three to four weeks until it's time to flip over to chapter 5 (when your baby is about six months old).

When you're ready for more intensity (and on days when baby happily acquiesces to a longer routine), repeat your workout a second time (or try both Routines 1 and 2 back-to-back) to create eighteen minutes of total-body exercise.

EXERCISE GUIDELINES FOR THIS CHAPTER

Read the steps below for what to expect from the workout in this chapter.

- Aim to do each strength exercise for forty-five to sixty seconds.

- For Routine 2, use hand weights between five and ten pounds (2.3–4.5kg). You should be lifting enough weight to make your working muscles feel fatigued by about forty-five to sixty seconds.

- For Routine 1, refer to the Intensity Boost sections for guidance on adding variety and intensity to some of the exercises.

- See the Trainer Tip in both routines to ensure that you get the most out of every move.

- As in the last chapter, there are C-section modifications for new moms who need them, but only for the moves in Routine 1. By the time most women who've had a cesarean reach four months postpartum (which is right around the time you'll be ready to try Routine 2), special modifications are no longer required.

- Do one or more of the nine-minute routines in this chapter every other day (or as close to that schedule as possible from week to week). This works out to be three to four times a week.

- Refer back to pages 22 and 23 in chapter 3 for instructions on how to fit "The Basic Three" exercises into your day.

- Check out the sidebar on pages 57 and 58 for a cardio workout you can do with a stroller or while wearing your baby.

- Finally, see pages 106 to 116 for stretches you can do after your workout, or whenever you can squeeze them in throughout the day.

Toe Taps with Punches and Half-Squats

Do it for: three minutes total

Minutes 1 and 2:
Toe taps with punches

1. Place your baby on the floor in front of you.

2. Stand with your feet wider than your hips and your arms by your sides.

3. Lift the heel on your right foot, tapping your toe on the right and bending both your knees slightly as you tap.

4. As you toe-tap on the right, rotate your right shoulder slightly toward the left.

5. Switch sides; tapping your left toe while rotating your left shoulder toward the right.

6. Alternate for thirty seconds, and then bend your elbows, tucking your forearms and hands into your chest in a boxer's stance.

When you toe-tap on your right, extend your right arm at shoulder height, rotating in a punch motion toward the left; repeat on the other side.

Minute 3:
Half-squats

1. Step forward so your feet are straddled on either side of your baby, with your toes facing forward and your ankles in line with your baby's ankles.

2. Reposition your feet to hip-width apart, then bend your legs to about forty-five degrees, lowering into a half-squat.

3. Keep your weight in your heels and avoid pushing your knees toward your toes.

4. Use your fingers to make tickling gestures at your baby (you probably won't be able to reach him without rounding your back, which is something you want to avoid).

Lunges

Works: legs, buttocks

Making It Work with Baby: Hold your baby facing forward or nestled into your chest, depending on what's most comfortable for both of you. Either way, your baby will enjoy the up-and-down motion as you complete each lunge.

C-Section Considerations: If you have trouble staying steady during lunges, rest your baby on the floor or cuddle him in one arm so you can balance yourself with one hand using a high-backed chair or crib.

🌸 TRAINER TIP

*The idea behind lunges is to move **down,** not forward. To get the right form, imagine that your back knee is being gently pulled toward the floor by a magnet while your front knee stays in line with your front ankle.*

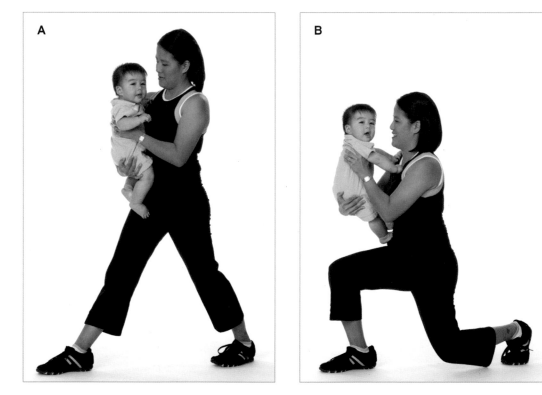

A. Stand with your feet hip-width apart, holding your baby in your arms or in a front carrier. Step your left foot behind you, balancing on the ball of your left foot and keeping your left heel off the floor. The toes on both feet should face forward.

B. Lower your left (back) knee toward the floor until both legs are bent at a ninety-degree angle. Keep your shoulders aligned over your hips (avoid leaning forward) and your belly button drawn toward your spine.

Return to the starting position and repeat for thirty seconds. Then switch sides, so your right foot is behind you. Do this for another thirty seconds on the other side.

Plié-Squats

Works: thighs, buttocks

Making It Work with Baby: Align your heels at your baby's ankles so she can easily look up at your face. Delight her by wiggling your fingers or dangling an eye-catching toy in the air as you lift your hands and arms with each plié-squat.

C-Section Considerations: If you find it difficult to balance, avoid standing directly over your baby; hold on to a sturdy piece of furniture to steady yourself.

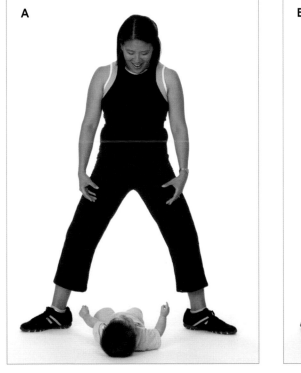

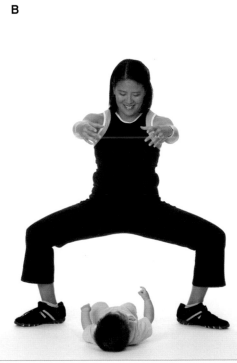

🌸 TRAINER TIP

Use visualization to really work your inner thighs. Here's how: As you straighten your legs from the Plié-Squat position, visualize gently squeezing your baby with your heels. Think of it as using your heels to hug your baby. Repeat this imaginary heel-hug every time you return to standing from the Plié-Squat.

◎ INTENSITY BOOST

Pick up your baby, holding her facing forward or into your chest. Her weight adds extra resistance to make you work harder.

A. Place a small blanket on the floor and lay your baby on her back. Stand in a plié position with feet wider than your shoulders. Your feet should be on either side of your baby but off the blanket for safety. Imagine a large clock underneath you as you turn your toes out to the ten o'clock and two o'clock positions.

B. With abdominals engaged, slowly bend your legs, as you raise your arms in front of you to just below shoulder height. Stop when your knees are aligned over your ankles and your thighs and arms are parallel to the floor. Return to standing as you lower your arms to your sides. Repeat.

Two-Legged Standing Calf Raises

Works: back of lower legs

Making It Work with Baby: Holding your baby adds extra resistance for developing strong, shapely lower legs. However, if your baby is fussing or isn't easily held with just one arm, lay her in her crib. Use the crib for support during these calf raises.

C-Section Considerations: To speed up your recovery and help flatten your belly, practice the Tummy Tuck move on page 22 during each calf raise.

TRAINER TIP
The object you choose for a balance support should be high enough to encourage you to stand tall and lengthen your spine without stooping over to reach it.

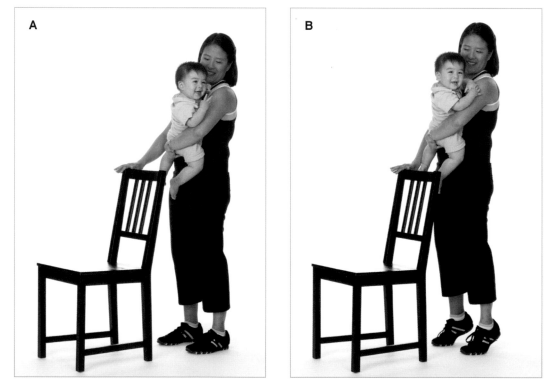

A. Stand next to a sturdy high-backed chair, crib, or change-table to use as a balance support. Hold your baby, facing in or out, with one arm. Place your free hand on the support object.

B. Position your feet hip-width apart, and then slowly raise both heels off the floor. Balance for one to two seconds on your toes. Slowly return both heels to the floor. Repeat.

Kiss-Your-Baby Push-ups

Works: chest, shoulders, arms

Making It Work with Baby: Baby lies on his back, gazing up at you. Position his head so it's directly under yours. If you lay your baby on a blanket, make sure the blanket isn't under your palms during the push-ups, which could cause your hands to slide.

C-Section Considerations: If you feel discomfort around your incision, try keeping your hips slightly elevated during this exercise (see Kiss-Your-Baby Push-ups in chapter 3).

A. With your baby lying faceup on the floor, get into a push-up position with your spine straight (avoid rounding your back) and your knees on the floor, feet in air. Place your hands on the floor about shoulder-width apart and on either side of baby.

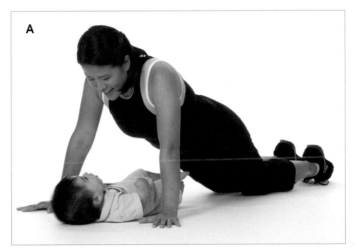

B. Look into your baby's face and bend your arms to the sides, lowering your face and chest toward the floor while keeping your back and neck straight. Kiss your baby! Straighten your arms to return to the starting position. Repeat.

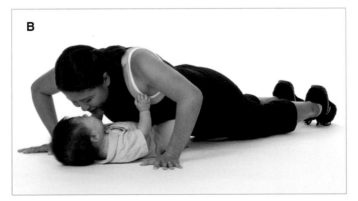

🌸 TRAINER TIP

Avoid straining your neck to reach your baby for a kiss. Use your chest and arm muscles to lower yourself toward your baby, keeping good form in your neck and back.

◎ INTENSITY BOOST

When your arms are bent to about ninety degrees, lift your right knee off the floor. Hold for three seconds, maintaining balance, before returning your right knee to the floor. Lift your left knee; hold for three seconds; lower your left knee to the floor. Avoid lifting your knee too high, which may strain your lower back. Return to the push-up starting position. If you have trouble staying steady on one knee, avoid this variation until you have full control of your balance.

Abdominal Planks

Works: abs, back

Making It Work with Baby: Make sure your baby's head is under yours so you can make eye contact. With your forearms on the floor, rest your palms near your baby's head; entertain or soothe her with tiny tickles.

C-Section Considerations: Keep your knees on the floor—forfeiting the more intense on-your-toes option described below—if you feel discomfort or tightness around your incision.

TRAINER TIP

A common technique problem with the plank is dropping your head toward the floor; maintaining face-to-face interaction with your baby ensures good form. To protect your lower back, avoid lowering your hips too close to the floor.

INTENSITY BOOST

To make this ab exercise harder, lift your knees off the floor, straightening your legs. Balance on your forearms and toes to create a straight line from your head to your legs.

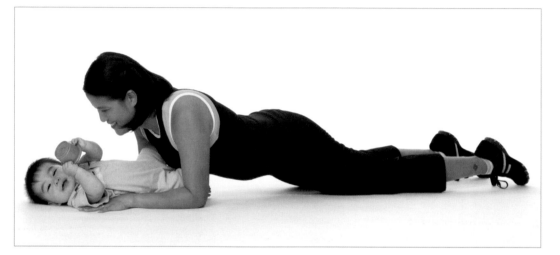

Rest baby on her back. Lie facedown with your forearms on either side of your baby, and shoulders and hips off the floor. Bend your hips slightly. Align your elbows under your shoulders.

Now tighten your abs as you release the bend in your hips, creating a diagonal line from your knees to the back of your head. Balance on your forearms and knees, feet touching the floor.

Hold for twenty-five seconds; rest for ten seconds; repeat for another twenty-five seconds.

Bridges

Works: buttocks, back of thighs, lower back

Making It Work with Baby: Your baby sits on your pelvis with his back supported by the front of your thighs. His legs can be straight and resting on your stomach, or straddled on either side of your pelvis, depending on your baby's size and what's most comfortable. Hold your baby's hands or grasp him around his hips or waist to keep him secure.

C-Section Considerations: If sitting your baby on your pelvis bothers your incision, place him on the floor or higher up your torso on your stomach.

A. Roll onto your back with your legs bent and the soles of your feet on the floor, heels about twelve inches (30.5cm) from your buttocks. Hold your baby, seated, on your pelvis.

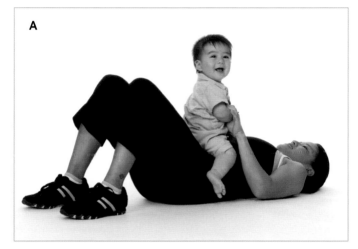

🌸 TRAINER TIP

Protect your back: Raise your hips to where you can comfortably hold your spine straight without overarching it. Squeeze your buttocks muscles to get the most out of this exercise. This also prevents your lower spine from dipping toward the floor and your pelvis from tilting side to side.

B. Slowly raise your hips off the floor, squeezing your buttocks muscles and keeping your spine straight (not curving in or out). Your feet, shoulder blades, and head remain on the floor. Hold this bridge position for three seconds before lowering your hips back to the floor. Repeat until the end of forty-five to sixty seconds.

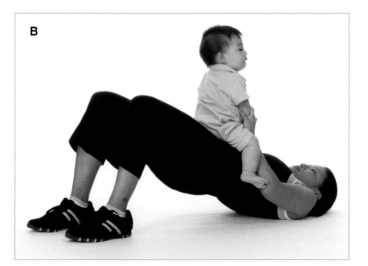

◎ INTENSITY BOOST

While your hips are raised, lift one heel (but not the toes) off the floor. Lower your heel as you return to the starting position. Raise your hips and repeat the heel lift on the other side. Alternate heel lifts.

Pelvic Tilt

Works: lower abs

Making It Work with Baby: Place your baby on the floor, in a supported chair, or against a sturdy pillow next to you.

C-Section Considerations: If your incision is still sensitive to touch, visualize a triangle (see below) instead of placing your hands on your pelvis.

TRAINER TIP

Avoid squeezing your butt muscles or lifting your hips off the floor during this exercise. Focus on using your abs to make your pelvis tilt forward and back.

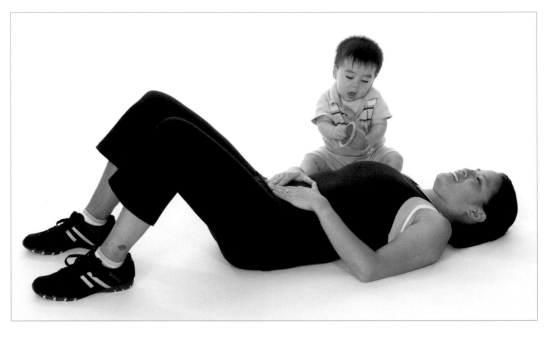

Lie on your back with your knees bent and your feet on the floor about hip-width apart. Place your thumbs and index (pointer) fingers together to form a triangle shape with your hands. Then place the "triangle" on the front of your pelvis with your thumbs just below your belly button. Imagine there's a marble in the center of the "triangle."

Then tilt your pelvis forward so your lower back lifts slightly off the floor. Visualize the imaginary marble rolling toward your pointer fingers.

Using your abs, tilt your pelvis back so your lower back touches the floor. Imagine the marble rolling toward your thumbs. Repeat this sequence.

Baby Chest Presses

Works: chest, shoulders, arms

Making It Work with Baby: Hold your baby with both your hands under her armpits and around her torso, your palms facing each other. As you lift your baby, keep her aligned over your chest and look into her face. Oh, and watch out for drool or spit-up bombs!

C-Section Considerations: Avoid placing your baby where she might accidentally kick your incision with her tiny feet.

A. Lie faceup with your baby on her tummy and lying on your chest. Bend your legs, placing the soles of your feet on the floor to support your back.

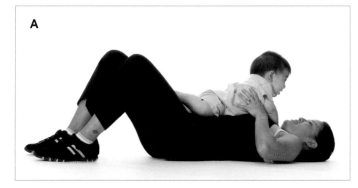

🐣 TRAINER TIP

If your baby is too heavy to comfortably lift in this position or she doesn't enjoy the sensation, you can work the same muscles with an extra set of Kiss-Your-Baby Push-ups instead.

B. Keeping your back and head on the floor, tighten your abs. Gently lift your baby in the air, until your arms are straight without locking your elbows, as shown. Slowly return your baby to your chest. Repeat for up to sixty seconds, depending on how long your baby enjoys the "ride."

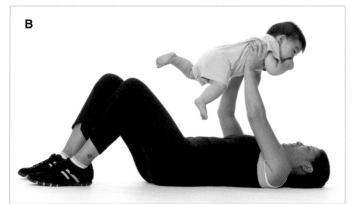

Airplane

Works: lower abs, back

Making It Work with Baby: With your baby supported against the front of your thighs, hold your baby's hands to the sides so he can have fun flying like an airplane as you extend your legs. Aviation sound effects optional.

C-Section Considerations: Keep your head on the floor; use a thin pillow or a folded blanket to prop up your head for a better view of your baby. If your incision is irritated by the weight of your baby, move her to the side for "tummy time" next to you.

✿ TRAINER TIP

If your neck muscles get too tired or feel strained, continue this exercise with your head resting on the floor. Use a firm pillow or a folded blanket for support.

◎ INTENSITY BOOST

Place your baby on your shins during Airplane so she can "fly" (baby is on her tummy). Be careful not to extend your legs to the point that your low abs pooch out or press into your hands.

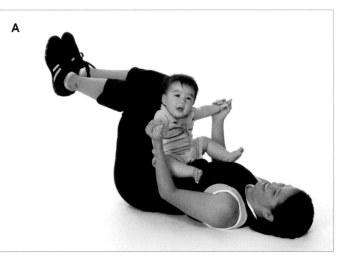

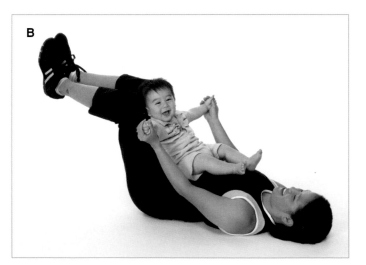

A. Lie on your back with your legs bent to ninety degrees, feet in air and hips in line with your knees. Place your baby on your lower abdomen. Hold both your baby's hands, with his arms to the sides. Or, if your neck gets tired, use just one hand to secure your baby's back against your legs and place your other hand behind your head to support your head and neck.

B. Lift your head slightly off the floor as you tighten your abs. Slowly extend your legs until your knees have moved about four to six inches (10–15cm) away from their original position. To avoid letting your lower belly pooch outward, keep your deep ab muscles (transverse abdominis) engaged, using the Tummy Tuck technique on page 22. Return to the starting position with your knees in line with your hips. Repeat.

Single-Arm Upright Rows

Works: back of shoulders, midback

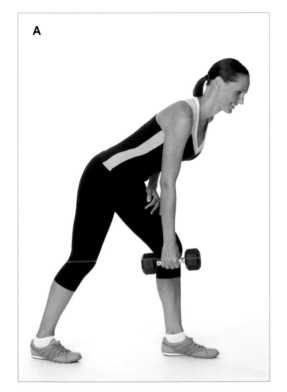

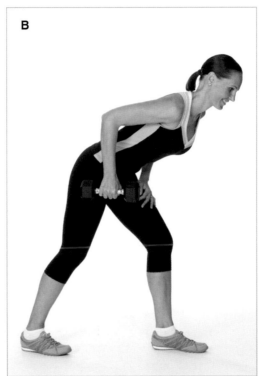

Keep the hand weight and your elbow close to your side as you lift the weight. Your elbow should be pointing behind you, not to the side, and your upper arm should be parallel to the floor at the top of the movement (i.e., right before you lower your arm to the starting position).

A. Hold a hand weight in your right hand, palm facing your body. Step your left foot slightly forward.

B. With your abs contracted, bend slightly forward from your waist, keeping your spine long and flat (avoid rounding your back). Lightly place your left hand on your left thigh for support. Align the hand weight under your right shoulder. Then lift the weight to the side of your ribcage, bending your elbow behind you. Repeat the movement for about thirty seconds; switch sides.

Shoulder Presses

Works: shoulders

TRAINER TIP

Avoid bending your wrists or arching your back.

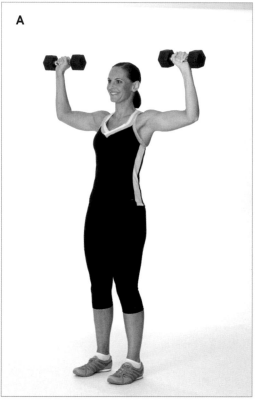

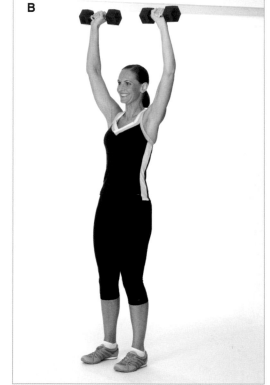

A. With one weight in each hand, bring the hand weights to shoulder height with arms bent. Your palms should face forward with your elbows pointing to the floor.

B. Raise your arms overhead until they are straight and your hands are aligned over your shoulders. Lower your arms until they are in line with your shoulders to return to starting position. Repeat.

Squats with Hip Extensions

Works: thighs, butt

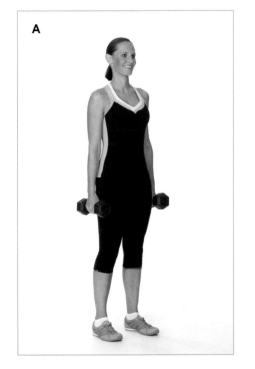

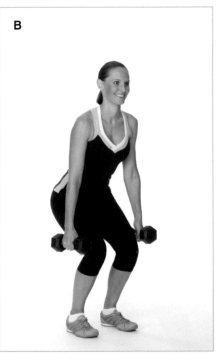

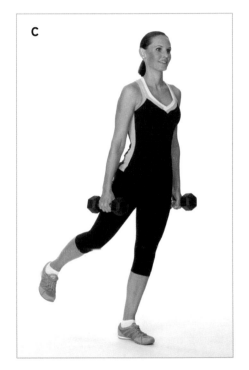

A. Stand with your feet hip-width apart and a hand weight in each hand. Your arms should be at your sides.

B. Slowly lower yourself into a squat as if you were sitting down on a chair behind you.

C. As you return to the standing position, lift your right foot off the floor and extend your right leg behind you, contracting your right butt muscle. Be careful not to lift your back leg too high in the air, which may strain the low back.

Lower your right foot to the starting position, squat again, and then extend your left leg behind you. Repeat the sequence.

🌸 TRAINER TIP

Make sure that your knees don't push past your toes as you squat down.

Biceps Curls (see page 98)

Works: front of the upper arms

1. Stand with your feet hip-width apart, holding a weight in each hand, arms at your sides and palms facing forward.
2. Bend both your arms to lift the weights toward your shoulders. Keep your elbows close to the body.
3. Extend your arms, lowering the weights to the starting position. Repeat.

One-Legged Lunges with Knee Lifts

Works: thighs, buttocks

🌸 TRAINER TIP

Biceps Curls: Keep your abs tight and your knees slightly bent throughout the biceps curls.

🌸 TRAINER TIP

One-Legged Lunge with Knee Lift: If doing the knee lift causes you to lose balance, put one hand weight down and use your free hand to steady yourself against the back of a chair or another sturdy piece of furniture.

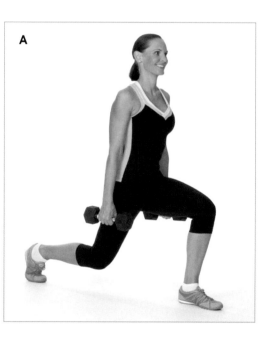

A. Start with feet hip-width apart and a hand weight in each hand. Step your right foot behind you into a lunge position; right heel is up.

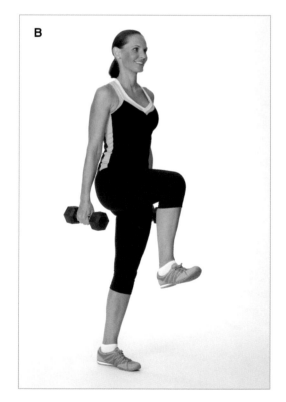

B. Lower your right (back) knee toward the floor. As you raise yourself out of the lunge, press off your back foot, bringing your right leg in front of your body, bent to ninety degrees. Immediately return to the lunge position by stepping your right foot behind you again, lowering your right knee toward the floor. Repeat the sequence for thirty seconds; switch sides.

Overhead Triceps Extensions

Works: back of the upper arms

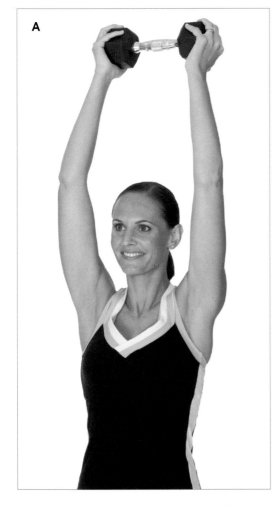

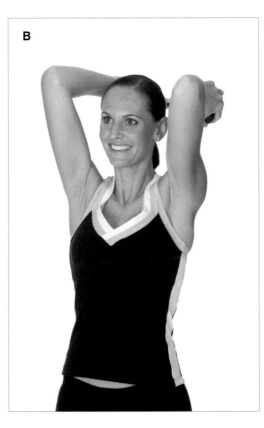

🌸 TRAINER TIP

Make sure your elbows are pointing upward, not directly to the sides.

B. Bend your arms, lowering the weight behind your head while keeping your upper arms close to your ears, as shown. Straighten your arms to the starting position. Repeat.

A. Grasp one of your heavy weights with both hands, or hold two light weights, one in each hand. Reach your arms overhead, holding the hand weight(s) either vertical or horizontal to the floor.

Side Planks with Arm Raises

Works: abs (obliques), back, shoulders

🌼 TRAINER TIP

If the shoulder exercise interferes with your good form during the side plank, eliminate the arm movement until you feel stronger.

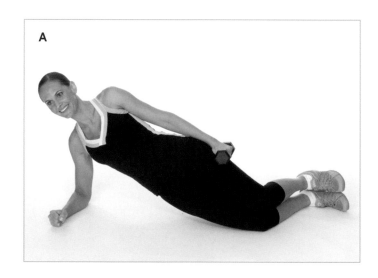

A. Lie on your right side with your right hip and forearm on the floor and legs bent so your feet are behind you. With your left arm at your side, hold a light hand weight in your left hand.

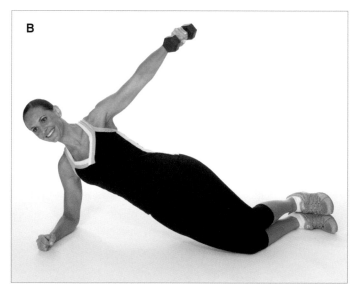

B. Contract your abs and lift your right hip off the floor, balancing yourself on your right forearm and the side of your right knee. From this position, slowly raise your left (top) arm until it's almost perpendicular to the floor (vertical). Return the arm to its starting position and repeat as you continue to hold yourself in a side plank. Do this exercise for thirty seconds; switch sides.

Chest Flyes

Works: arms, shoulders, chest

A. Lie faceup with your knees bent, feet flat on the floor. Holding a hand weight in each hand, straighten your arms upward so they are aligned over your chest. Your palms should be facing each other.

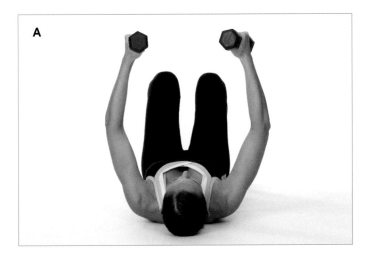

TRAINER TIP

Contract your abs to help protect your back; avoid arching your spine as you lower the hand weights.

B. Keeping your elbows slightly bent, slowly lower your arms to the sides until the hand weights are just above your shoulders on either side.

Return to the starting position, maintaining the slight bend in your elbows. Repeat.

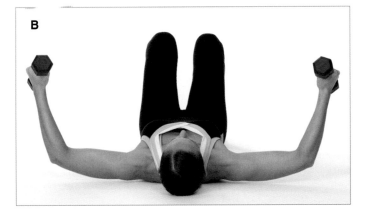

Heel Slides with Weights

Works: upper and lower abs

🌼 TRAINER TIP

If you have difficulty keeping your abs properly contracted, put the hand weight down and try this exercise with your arms and hands on the floor for support.

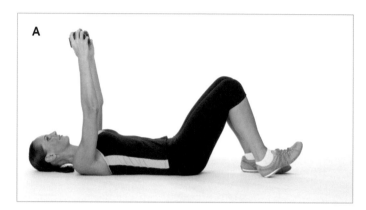

A. Lie faceup with knees bent, feet flat on the floor. Holding one hand weight with both hands, extend your arms in the air so the hand weight is aligned over your chest and horizontal to the floor.

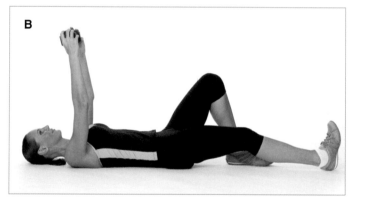

B. Contract your abs and slowly slide your right foot away from your buttocks until that moving leg is almost straight. Return your foot to the starting position. Repeat on your left side.

38-Minute Cardio Workout

Do this cardio workout three to four times a week with your baby in a stroller or front carrier. Check that you are at the right intensity with the

• "talk test" (you should be able to comfortably speak to your baby without gasping for air).

• the Rating of Perceived Exertion (RPE) chart on page 34 (chapter 3).

What You Need
• supportive shoes
• water bottle
• your baby in a stroller or front carrier
• a watch that shows time in seconds

Warm-Up

Do it for: five minutes

Walk at a moderate pace, taking long steps to lengthen your hip flexor muscles and raise your body's temperature. As you walk, roll your shoulders back and down for good posture. Push off the ball of your foot with each step.

Drill 1: Thirty/Thirty-Second Intervals

Do it for: fourteen minutes

Interval A: Walk at a challenging pace for thirty seconds, moving fast but taking short steps. Your RPE should be 6.

Interval B: Walk for another thirty seconds at a slower pace, still using short strides; walk on your toes to work your calves. Your RPE should be 5.

Alternate Intervals A and B for fourteen minutes, and then try Drill 2 (see page 58).

Tip for walking with a stroller: Keep your wrists straight and your hips facing the stroller's handlebars.

Tip for walking with a carrier: Your upper back and shoulders are prone to slouch forward from carrying your baby at the front of your body. The fix? Keep your abs contracted as much as possible and stand with your chest open. Avoid pushing your belly out to support your baby.

Drill 2: Forty-Five/Fifteen-Second Intervals

Do it for: fourteen minutes

Interval C: Walk for forty-five seconds at a challenging pace, moving quickly and with slightly longer steps to rev up your heart rate and challenge your leg muscles even more. Your RPE should be 7.

Interval D: Slow down for fifteen seconds to recover from Interval C. Walk at a moderate pace. Your RPE should be 5.

Alternate Intervals C and D for fourteen minutes.

Tip for walking with a stroller: Avoid leaning forward at the waist and pushing the stroller away from you as you go uphill or begin to get tired; stay close to your baby!

Tip for walking with a carrier: When doing intervals that could make your legs tired, walk on even, flat terrain for better balance.

Cooldown

Do it for: five minutes

Walk at an easy pace, switching between short steps for one minute and long steps for one minute.

Extending the Workout
After four weeks: Do a 45-minute cardio.* Complete Drills 1 and 2, and then repeat Drill 1 for seven minutes.

After eight weeks: Do a fifty-two-minute cardio.* Complete Drills 1 and 2, and then repeat Drill 1 for fourteen minutes.

*This includes five minutes of warm-up and five minutes of cooldown

CHAPTER 5

Your Baby Is Six to Eight Months Old

When you were still pregnant, you might have imagined that by the time your baby turned half a year old, your body would be right back to its prepregnancy shape. Maybe you anticipated that you'd be slipping into your favorite pair of before-baby jeans by now. Or that any unwanted "baby fat" would be gone when six months postpartum rolled around. It does happen this way for some new moms (if you're one of them, keep reading—building muscular strength and stamina is still important). But for most of us? Well, we have to be patient. The majority of women with six-month-old babies still have at least some pregnancy weight to lose. So store your "skinny jeans" in the closet for just a little longer.

That's not to say there hasn't been progress. If you've been following the exercises in this book and eating well so far, you've likely shed pounds. And your arms and legs probably look and feel firmer. I suspect that you've also noticed that your ab strength is a lot better, compared to just a few months ago. However, if you feel as if the skin on your tummy is still softer or looser than you'd like, don't be discouraged. That'll eventually firm up, too, with regular exercise.

It's not uncommon for new moms to feel as if they've hit a fat-loss or fitness plateau around this time. To bust past such a plateau, be as consistent as possible with exercise so you're able to safely and realistically intensify your workouts.

Ready to try a couple of new routines? The moves on the following pages were designed for your postpartum body as it is now. Plus, the exercise-with-baby workout (Routine 1) takes into account what your little one might be up to these days.

What's Happening, Baby?

At around this time your baby is probably able to sit up on his own, which makes it easier for you to do the exercises in this chapter without your having to keep one hand free to prop him up. Babies at around this age also roll from their back to their tummy, and vice versa. So if you place baby on the floor, be extra mindful about where he is underfoot before stepping forward, back, or to the sides during the warm-up routine and exercises such as alternating lunges.

Now is the time when you'll be introducing your baby to solid foods. In a month or two, your infant may be holding and munching

WHAT YOU'RE LIFTING THESE DAYS: YOUR BABY'S WEIGHT		
WEEKS	**WEIGHT**	**DATE**
30-31		
32-33		
34-35		
36-37		
38-39		
40-41		
42-43		

baby-friendly crackers or similar snacks all on her own. This new-to-her activity might spare you just enough time to zip through the nine-minute hand-weight workout (Routine 2) in this chapter. Why not settle her into a high chair (or another locale where you can supervise) and see what happens? Otherwise, consider scheduling your workout during naptime or when backup—a babysitter, your partner, grandma—comes to the rescue.

By month six or seven, you may notice that your baby likes to reach for toys. To keep her busy, pass new or favorite toys or objects to her as you exercise.

By eight months old, your baby may be moving from one spot to another. If you find yourself chasing a roller or beginner-crawler, while also trying desperately to get through an exercise routine, don't get frustrated. Consider the extra calorie-burning activity part of your workout. Tip: Remember to baby-proof the area where you'll be exercising beforehand so you don't have to keep stopping midworkout to secure a cupboard door or scoop up stuff you don't want your baby to get her hands on.

One last comment about your baby's development: By now, he may have more than doubled his birth weight. He's getting heavier by the week, and you might find that using a front carrier is just not comfortable anymore. Exercising while holding your baby will become more challenging. That's good news for your muscles, which need to be challenged in order get stronger and firmer. But to prevent injury, I encourage you to keep doing "The Basic Three" exercises in chapter 3, pages 22 and 23 (of course, you've been faithfully doing them all along . . . right?).

Read on for tips about what to expect from the workouts in this chapter.

How to Get Started

The two whole-body workouts on the following pages are more intense than in the previous chapters. Try Routine 1 for about three weeks. Then do Routine 2 for the next three weeks. After that, switch between the two nine-minute routines on the following pages every three weeks until you reach about eight months postpartum. Note that Routine 2 requires you to use hand weights for resistance instead of your baby's weight.

When you're ready for more intensity or actually have a little extra time on your hands, repeat your workout a second time (or do Routine 1 followed by Routine 2). Then pat yourself on the back for squeezing in a full-body workout in just nine to eighteen minutes.

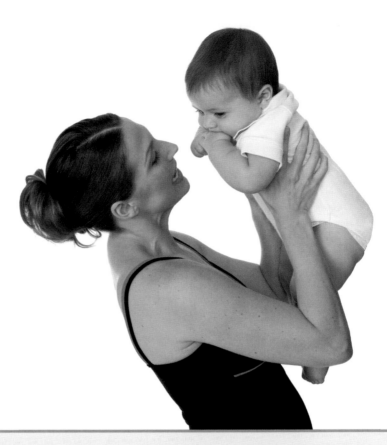

EXERCISE GUIDELINES FOR THIS CHAPTER

Read the steps below for what to expect from the
workout in this chapter.

• Each strength exercise should last for about forty-five to
sixty seconds. Lift heavy enough hand weights in
Routine 2 (I suggest between five and ten pounds
[2.3–4.5kg]) to adequately challenge your muscles
within this time frame.

• Refer to the Intensity Boost tips in Routine 1 if you want
to make an exercise harder or just a little different.

• Make your workouts as safe and effective as possible by
reading the Trainer Tips that accompany each exercise.

• Unlike the previous chapters, you won't find C-section
modifications here; by six months postpartum, you
should no longer need exercise modifications. If you
continue to feel discomfort at your point of incision with
any exercises, stop exercising and consult your physician or midwife as soon as possible.

• Do one or more of the nine-minute routines in this
chapter on every other day (or as close to that schedule
as possible from week to week). This works out to be
three to four times a week.

• Follow the instructions at the end of this chapter for a
fat-blasting cardio workout, and see chapter 7 for
stretches you can do postexercise or whenever you have
a spare moment.

Knee Lifts and Side Squats

Do it for: three minutes total

Minute 1:
Knee lifts with arms reaching overhead

1. Place your baby on a blanket on the floor in front of you.

2. Stand with your feet hip-width apart.

3. Lift your right foot off the floor, bringing your right knee to hip height.

4. Lower your leg, and repeat on the left side. Alternate knee lifts.

5. Add arm movements: As you lift alternating knees, reach your arms overhead, aligning your hands over your shoulders, palms facing forward.

Minute 2:
Side squats with chest presses

1. Stand with feet together and arms bent at chest height, hands next to your shoulders and elbows pointing behind you.

2. Step your right foot to your right side as you bend your legs into a squat.

3. As you squat, straighten your arms in front of you in a "chest press" motion, palms facing the floor.

4. Return to the starting position.

5. Step your left foot to your left side. At the same time, bend your legs and squat; press your arms in front of you.

6. Return to the starting position and repeat.

Minute 3:
Knee lifts with arms reaching overhead

Repeat sequence from Minute 1 above.

Alternating Reverse Lunges

Works: legs, butt

Making It Work with Baby: Hold baby facing forward or looking over your shoulder. If you prefer less resistance or you need a free hand to balance yourself against a chair, crib, or wall, place baby on the floor. Make sure that he is far enough away from you so he doesn't roll underfoot while you're in motion.

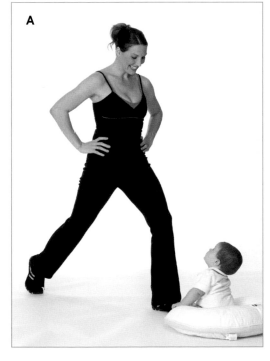

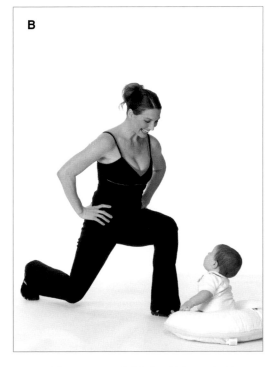

A. Stand with your feet hip-width apart, holding your baby in your arms (or see alternative above). Step your right foot behind you.

B. Next, lower your right (back) knee to the floor. You should be on the ball of your right foot with your right heel off the floor.

Return to the starting position, and then immediately perform a reverse lunge on the opposite side. Repeat the sequence, alternating reverse lunges.

✿ TRAINER TIP

Protect your back by keeping your abs tight and your shoulders aligned over your hips.

◎ INTENSITY BOOST

After each lunge and before you bring your feet together, straighten your back leg, lifting your back foot off the floor. At the same time, squeeze your buttocks muscle on the same side as the lifted leg (i.e., contract your right butt muscle when your right leg is extended behind you). Avoid lifting your leg too high; do a small lift and squeeze. Return to the starting position and repeat on the other side.

Squats with Gentle Baby Lifts

Works: thighs, buttocks, shoulders, arms

Making It Work with Baby: As you lift and lower your baby, repeat the words up and down to teach your baby the corresponding directions and keep her entertained. If lifting your baby and squatting at the same time feels too intense, just cuddle her at chest level.

TRAINER TIP

To guard against back and shoulder strain, avoid raising your baby more than a few inches higher than your shoulders.

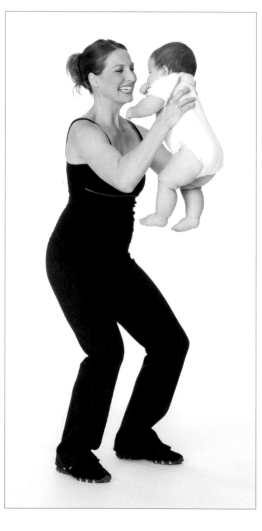

Place your feet slightly wider than hip-width apart, toes facing forward, and hold your baby against your chest. With abs engaged, bend your legs, lowering yourself into a squat position until your knees are aligned over your ankles. As you squat, slowly lift your baby upwards about six inches (15cm).

Return to standing and lower your baby, snuggling her into your chest. Repeat.

Kiss-Your-Baby Straight-Leg Push-ups

Works: chest, shoulders, arms, thighs, abs

Making It Work with Baby: A month or two ago, your baby lay stationary on his back as you did from-the-knees push-ups. Now you're stronger (hence the from-the-toes push-ups) and so is he. At this stage, he may want to roll this way and that, bumping into your arms as you lower yourself down and up. Alternative position for baby: Sit him in front of you so you can kiss his tiny toes, midpush-up.

A. Get into a push-up position with your back straight (not rounded), legs straight, and toes on floor. Your feet should be about hip-width apart. Place your hands on the floor slightly wider than shoulder-width apart and on either side of baby, who is lying faceup on the floor.

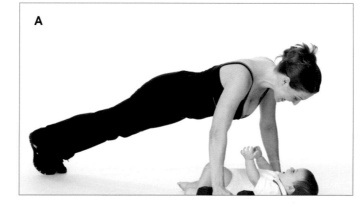

B. Look into your baby's face and bend your arms to the sides, lowering your face, chest, and pelvis toward the floor while keeping your back and neck straight. Kiss your baby!

Straighten your arms to return to the starting position. Repeat for up to sixty seconds (see Trainer Tip box).

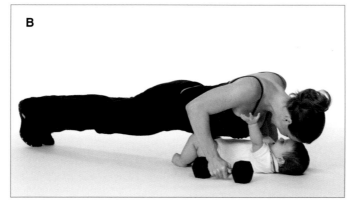

🌸 TRAINER TIP

Doing push-ups from your toes is no easy feat. If it feels too hard to go a full minute like this, attempt twenty seconds of straight-leg push-ups, then lower onto your knees for the final forty seconds. From there, gradually increase the time you spend doing the straight-leg version.

Abdominal Planks on Toes

Works: abs, back, thighs

Making It Work with Baby: Make sure your baby's head is under yours so you can make eye contact. With your forearms on the floor, rest your palms on baby's head—entertain or soothe her with tiny tickles. Or, let her practice rolling nearby.

🌸 TRAINER TIP

Balance your weight on your forearms and your toes, making sure your hips do not push toward the ceiling or drop toward the floor (i.e., maintain a straight line from your head to your heels).

🌀 INTENSITY BOOST

Lift your right foot off the floor, holding it in the air and contracting your right butt muscle for fifteen seconds. Release and switch sides, lifting your left foot off the floor for fifteen seconds. Repeat the sequence for a total of sixty seconds.

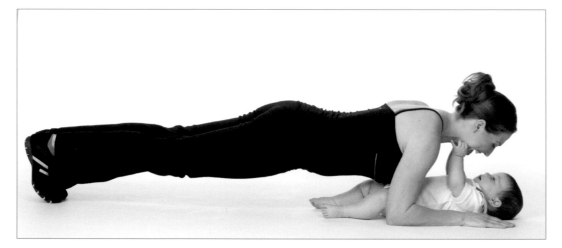

Rest baby on her back. Lie facedown with your forearms on either side of your baby, elbows under your shoulders. Your shoulders and hips are off the floor, and your knees and toes are touching the floor.

Tighten your abs as you lift your knees off the floor, straightening your legs. Your head, hips, and heels should be in line, as shown.

Hold the plank position for twenty-five seconds; rest for ten seconds; hold the plank position for another twenty-five seconds. Gradually work up to more plank time and less rest time.

Triceps Dips

Works: back of upper arms

Making It Work with Baby: Sit your baby between your feet so she can make eye contact and say "Hello" each time you lower your hips.

A. Sit on the floor with your feet hip-width apart and your palms flat on the floor slightly behind you, fingertips facing your feet. Your elbows should be slightly bent and pointing behind you. Slowly lift your hips off the floor until they are almost in line with your knees and shoulders.

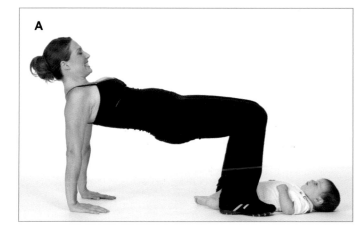

B. Bend your arms, keeping your elbows pointing behind you. Allow your buttocks to lower toward the floor without touching the floor, as shown.

Straighten your arms and lift your hips to complete one rep.

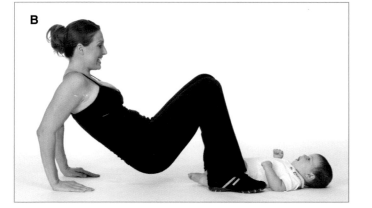

❀ TRAINER TIP

Keep your elbows moving back, behind your shoulders. It should feel as if you're squeezing your elbows together. If this move bothers your wrists, opt instead for the Kneeling Triceps Kickbacks in Routine 2 on page 76.

◎ INTENSITY BOOST

Lift one foot off the floor as you do the triceps dip. Alternate feet with each rep.

Side-Lying Leg Lifts

Works: hips, outer thighs

Making It Work with Baby: Place your baby on his back, side, or stomach next to you.

⚘ TRAINER TIP

Occasionally put your top hand on your abs as a reminder to keep them engaged. Angle your big toe on the top foot slightly toward the ground instead of the ceiling to work the muscles in your outer hip and thigh more effectively.

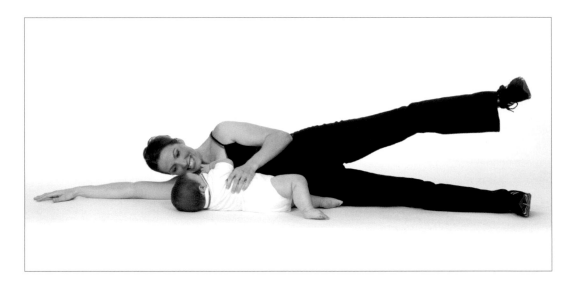

Lie on your right side with your hips and legs stacked one on top of the other. Extend your right arm so it's lying on the floor; rest the side of your head on that arm.

Lift your left leg about twelve to eighteen inches (30.5–45.5cm) into the air, as shown. Hold for two to three seconds. Lower your top (left) leg to the starting position. Repeat for twenty to thirty seconds. Switch sides.

Low Back Extensions

Works: low back

Making It Work with Baby: Place your baby next to you with toys to occupy her. Avoid looking up too high while you are in this position. Doing so may strain your neck. Interact with your baby, using your voice rather than eye contact. Say, "up" as you lift into the back extension and "down" as you lower yourself to the floor.

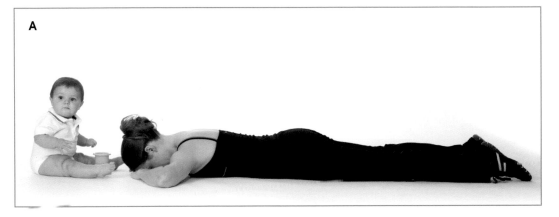

A

A. Lie facedown on the floor with your legs straight and your shoelaces (top of feet) facing the floor. Bend your arms so your elbows point to the sides. Place your hands under your forehead, palms facing the floor.

⚘ TRAINER TIP

Keep your feet on the floor throughout this exercise. Focus on lifting just your head and shoulders off the floor. Engage your abdominals throughout.

◎ INTENSITY BOOST

Reach your arms overhead to make this exercise harder.

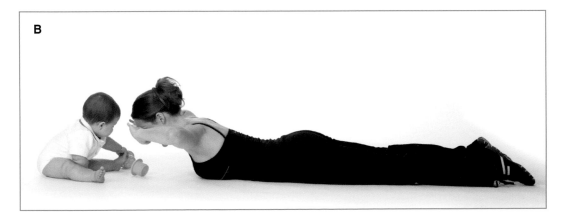

B

B. Gently lift your head and shoulders about four to six inches (10–15cm) off the floor. Lower your upper body back to the ground.

One-Side Oblique Crunches

Works: the ab muscles that wrap around your waist

Making It Work with Baby: Place your baby on the floor for tummy time so she can practice pushing up into a crawling position.

TRAINER TIP

Imagine reaching your finger tips toward your toes as you reach your top arm up and over. Move slowly and with control.

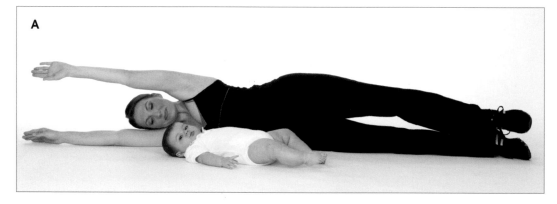

A. Lie on your side with your legs straight. Extend your arms overhead, placing your right palm flat on the floor.

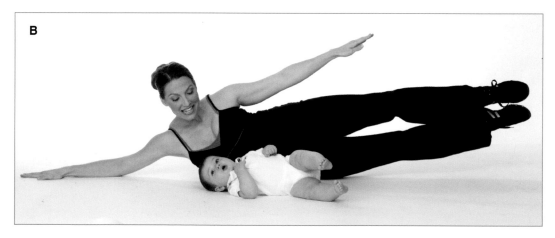

B. Lift your head and shoulders off the floor as you simultaneously lift both legs. Release and repeat for twenty to thirty seconds. Switch to the other side so that your left palm is flat on the floor and repeat for another twenty to thirty seconds.

Supine Toe Taps

Works: abs

Making It Work with Baby: Sit your baby on your hips/stomach so he's straddling your torso. Use one hand to keep him safely in place.

A. Lie on your back with your knees bent and your feet flat on the floor. Lift your legs into the air, keeping them bent to ninety degrees with your knees aligned over your hips.

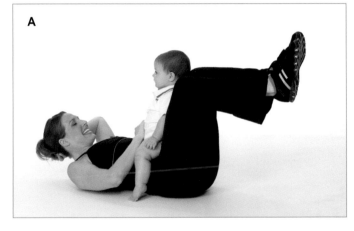

B. Draw your abs toward your spine as you lift your head off the floor, placing one hand behind your head for support. Slowly lower your right foot toward the floor without actually touching the floor.

Raise your right foot, bringing your right knee in line with your right hip. Repeat with your left leg, then alternate toe taps.

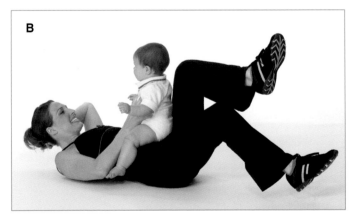

TRAINER TIP

If your lower spine arches toward the ceiling and your lower belly pooches outward, your abs may not be strong enough to complete this exercise yet. To modify it, shorten your range of motion by lowering your feet only halfway toward the floor before returning to the starting position. You may also rest your head on the floor.

INTENSITY BOOST

Instead of alternating toe taps, lower both feet toward the floor at the same time. To avoid straining your back, you may wish to reduce your range of motion (i.e., don't lower your feet all the way to the floor).

Lunges with Hammer Curls

Works: legs, butt, front of upper arms

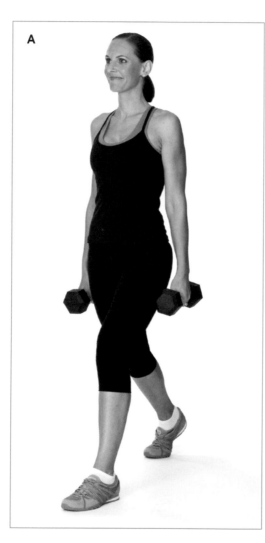

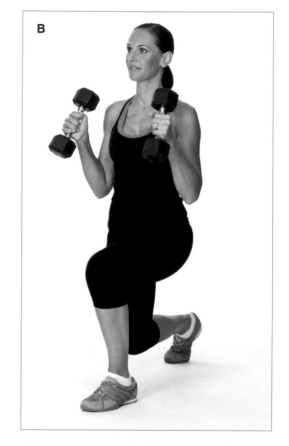

B. Lower your back (right) knee toward the floor into a lunge position. Simultaneously bend your arms, curling the hand weights toward your shoulders, palms still facing in, as shown.

A. Stand with your feet hip-width apart. Hold your hand weights, arms by your sides and palms facing toward your body. Step your right foot behind you, balancing on the ball of your right foot, heel off the floor.

Straighten your arms as you return to a standing position. Repeat for thirty seconds, then switch legs. (You may give your arms a short rest if you need to, but keep your legs moving.)

Reverse Flyes with Leg Lift

Works: back of shoulders, upper back, butt

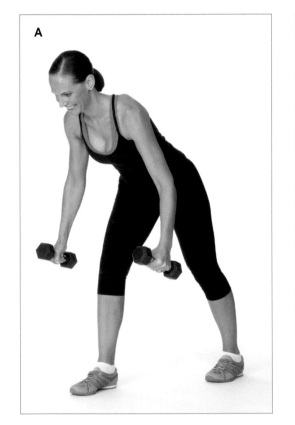

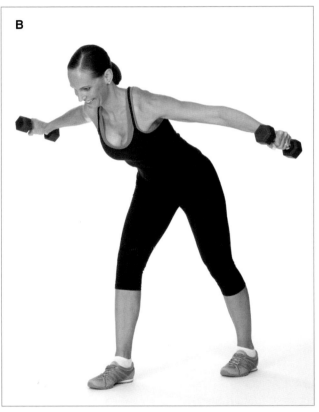

A. With one weight in each hand, stand with feet hip-width apart. Step one foot about eighteen inches (45.5cm) forward. Bend at the waist; keep your spine straight and hold your abs tight. Your arms should be at your sides, hands aligned under your shoulders.

B. With elbows slightly bent, raise your arms to the sides until your hands are just below shoulder height. At the same time, lift your back leg off the floor until your foot is almost level with your hip (not shown in photo). Slowly lower your foot to the floor and your hands to your sides. Repeat for thirty seconds; switch legs.

🏋 TRAINER TIP

Squeeze your shoulder blades together as you raise your arms.

One-Legged Squats with Shoulder Raises

Works: middle of shoulders, thighs, butt

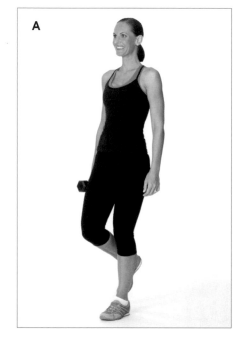

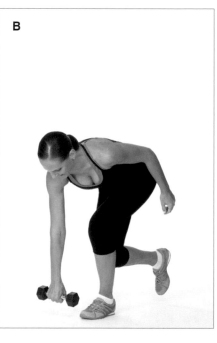

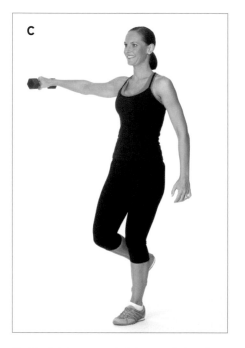

A. Hold one hand weight in your right hand. Stand with your feet hip-width apart, and then shift your weight to your left foot. Lift your right foot off the floor, balancing on your left leg, left knee slightly bent.

B. Bend your left leg into a one-legged squat as you also reach your right hand toward your left foot.

C. Straighten your left leg and simultaneously raise your right arm to your right side until the hand weight is just below shoulder height.

Return to the starting position and repeat for thirty seconds. Switch arm and leg.

🌸 TRAINER TIP

Make sure you bend your leg to bring yourself closer to the ground rather than bowing or leaning forward at the waist.

The Crawl

Works: arms, abs, thighs

A. Get into a straight-leg, push-up position while holding a hand weight in each hand, arms straight (the weights should be resting on the floor). Align your shoulders over your hands and place your feet hip-width apart. Your palms should be facing in toward each other.

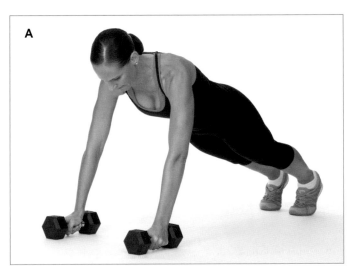

🌸 TRAINER TIP

Avoid pushing your hips up toward the ceiling. Keep your abs tight to protect your back and strengthen your core.

B. Contract your abs, lifting your right foot off the floor and bringing your right knee toward your chest, as shown.

Return your right foot to its starting position and repeat the movement with your left leg. Alternate sides.

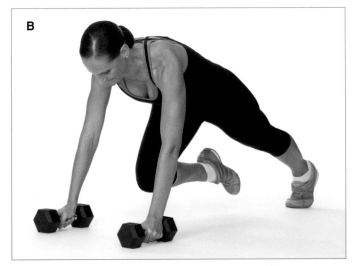

Kneeling Triceps Kickbacks

Works: back of upper arms

TRAINER TIP

Keep your elbow close to your side and your chest facing your thigh.

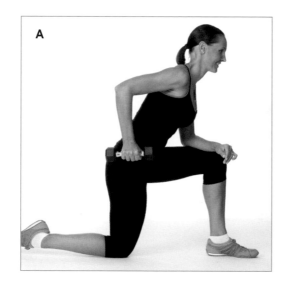

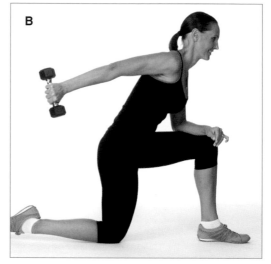

A. Place your left foot on the floor with your left knee bent and your right knee on the floor. Lightly place your left forearm on your left thigh, holding one hand weight in your right hand. Lean forward from your waist without rounding your back. Tighten your abs.

B. Lift your right elbow, bending your right arm until the weight is aligned under your right elbow. Straighten your right arm until it is parallel to the floor, squeezing the muscles in the back of your upper arm. Bend your arm and repeat for thirty seconds; switch sides.

Chest Presses

Works: chest, shoulders, arms

A. Lie on your back with your legs bent and your feet flat on the floor, hip-width apart. With a weight in each hand, straighten your arms so your hands are a little wider than shoulder-width apart, palms facing your knees.

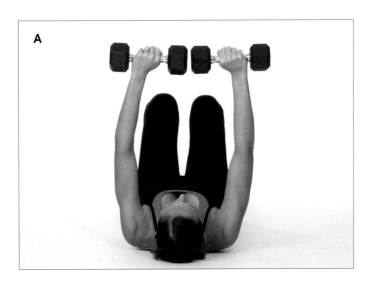

🌸 TRAINER TIP
Keep the weights aligned over your chest, not your face.

B. Slowly bend your arms, lowering the weights until your upper arms almost touch the floor. Your knuckles should be facing the ceiling, as shown. Slowly straighten your arms and repeat.

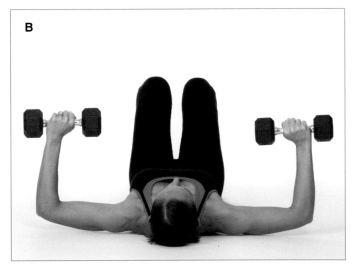

Side Planks with Rotator Cuff

Works: abs, shoulders

🌸 TRAINER TIP

Keep your shoulders in line so your chest faces forward, not toward the floor.

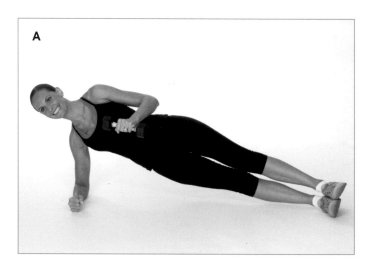

A. Lie on your right side with your right hip and forearm on the floor, right shoulder in line with right elbow. Hold a light weight in your left hand; bend your left arm so your forearm is parallel to the floor (palm faces floor), resting your elbow on your top hip. Stack your top foot on your bottom foot, as shown.

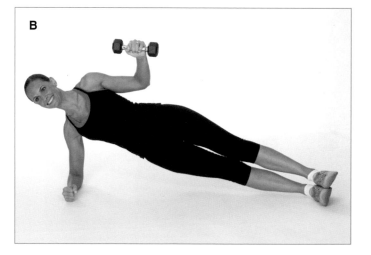

B. Lift your right hip off the floor, balancing on your forearm and your feet to hold your body in a diagonal line. At the same time, rotate through the top (left) shoulder, bringing your forearm up until your palm faces forward. Keep your top (left) elbow touching your body.

Return to the starting position and repeat for thirty seconds. Switch sides, lying on your left side with the weight in your right hand.

Side-Lying Leg Lifts with Shoulder Raises

Works: hips, outer thighs

A. Lie on your right side. Extend your right arm on the floor and use it as a headrest. Hold one light hand weight in your top (left) hand, placing your left hand on the side of your left thigh.

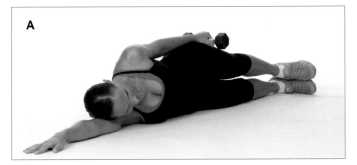

A

🏋 TRAINER TIP

Point the big toe on your top leg slightly toward the floor to really target the hip muscles during this exercise.

B. Lift your top (left) leg away from your bottom (right) leg. At the same time, raise your left arm about forty-five degrees in the air. Your right hip and right leg should stay on the floor, as shown.

Return your top leg to the starting position. Repeat for thirty seconds; switch sides.

B

Planks with Side-to-Side Toe Taps

Works: abs, arms, legs

TRAINER TIP

Keep your head and hips/butt aligned and avoid rounding or arching your back as your feet move from side to side.

A. Place hand weights out of the way and lie facedown with your forearms on the floor, elbows under shoulders. Your shoulders and hips should be off the floor with knees and toes touching the floor. Tighten your abs and raise your knees off the floor, straightening your legs.

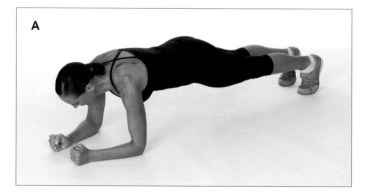

B. Slowly move your right foot about twelve inches (30.5cm) to your right, touching your right toes to the floor. Bring your right foot back to the starting position.

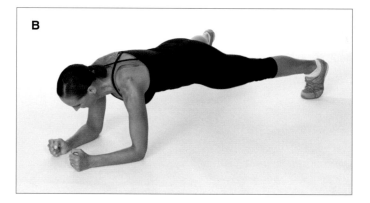

C. Move your left foot about twelve inches (30.5cm) to the left, tapping the floor with your left toes, as shown. Return to the starting position. Repeat sequence.

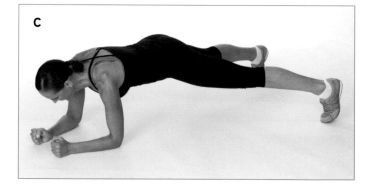

45-Minute Cardio Workout

Do this cardio workout four times a week with your baby in a stroller that you can jog or power-walk with. Check that you are at the right intensity with the

- "talk test" (you should be able to comfortably speak to your baby without gasping for air)

- the Rating of Perceived Exertion (RPE) chart on page 34

What You Need
- supportive shoes
- water bottle
- your baby in a jogging-style stroller (see Appendix B, pages 136 to 138, for tips on how to select a jogging-style stroller)
- a watch that shows time in seconds

Warm-Up

Do it for: five minutes

Walk at a moderate speed for the first two minutes (RPE: 3), and then gradually increase your pace until you're power-walking for the last minute of the warm-up (work up to RPE: 5).

Drill 1: Four/One-Minute Jog/Walk Intervals

Do it for: twenty minutes

Interval A: Jog at a comfortable but challenging pace for four minutes. If you prefer low-impact movement, substitute power walking instead of jogging. Your RPE should be 6.

Interval B: Walk at a moderate pace for one minute to recover from the jogging interval. Take long steps, striking the ground with your heel first, and then rolling onto your toes. Your RPE should be 3.

Alternate Intervals A and B for twenty minutes (four times total), and then try Drill 2 (see below).

Tip for walking with a jogging stroller: As you transition from walking to jogging, you might be tempted to hold the stroller away from your body and lean into it. To ensure good stroller-jogging (or power-walking) posture, keep the stroller close to your hips as opposed to pushing it with your arms extended.

Drill 2: Two/Two-Minute Jog/Walk Intervals

Do it for: sixteen minutes

Interval C: Jog (or power-walk) for two minutes at a challenging pace. This interval should feel as if you are going breathless by the end of the two minutes. Your RPE should be 7.

Interval D: Slow down to recover from Interval C. Walk at a moderate pace for two minutes. Your RPE should be 4–5.

Alternate Intervals C and D for sixteen minutes (four times total).

Tip for jogging with a stroller: Lower the handlebars during jogging intervals for easier pivoting of the stroller. Jog with one hand on the handlebar (with the safety strap around your wrist) and your other hand moving freely.

Cooldown

Do it for: four minutes

Stroll at a gentle pace to cool down (RPE: 3–4).

Extending the Workout
After four to eight weeks: For variety and to fast-track your fitness and/or weight-loss goals, do one additional cardio activity per week, such as swimming, cycling, or a fitness class.

CHAPTER 6

Your Baby Is Nine to Twelve Months Old

If you're reading this chapter when your baby is about nine or ten months old, you've now been not pregnant for as long as you were expecting! Nine months goes by in a flash, whether you're planning for the arrival of a newborn or getting to know the intricate needs and wants of the new little person in your life. By this point, you've come to recognize your baby's disposition, which makes it easier to keep her entertained. Is your baby the type to make a break for it, wriggling or crawling away to explore what's around her? Perhaps she's more prone to sit by your side, quietly studying a board book or tactile toy. Most babies tend to do a bit of both, depending on their mood.

Whether you already have two or more kids or you're a parent for the first time, you've likely learned that babies are unpredictable. Just when you think you have naptime running like clockwork, your baby decides he's done with a.m. snoozes. Or, you planned to have your baby well fed before your quickie afternoon workout, but he unexpectedly turns his nose up at your offering—pureed yams, a dish he normally relishes. Perhaps teething pain is making your baby especially cranky. What worked on Monday might not fly on Wednesday, right?

Still, there are glimpses of predictability! Knowing your baby's personality—outgoing or reserved—and sensing whether she's in the mood for an adventure or a cuddle helps you determine what to expect when you work out with your baby on any given day. This knowledge goes a long way toward creating an enjoyable experience for both of you.

In the chapters that follow, you'll find partner exercises you can do with another mom/baby duo, plus a strength workout for outdoors. This chapter, however, contains the last of the postpartum-specific nine-minute routines. So you have my congratulations! You've come a long way since the first chapters of this book, when you were recovering from childbirth and dealing with postural woes brought on by pregnancy and newborn care. If you've been following this book from the beginning, you're probably enjoying how your increasingly fit body looks and feels, no matter what your weight.

Take a moment to recognize the many fitness achievements you've reached as you progressed through each chapter of this book! Along the way, you've been demonstrating good exercise habits—ones that will make a lasting and positive impression on your child(ren). You may be nearing the

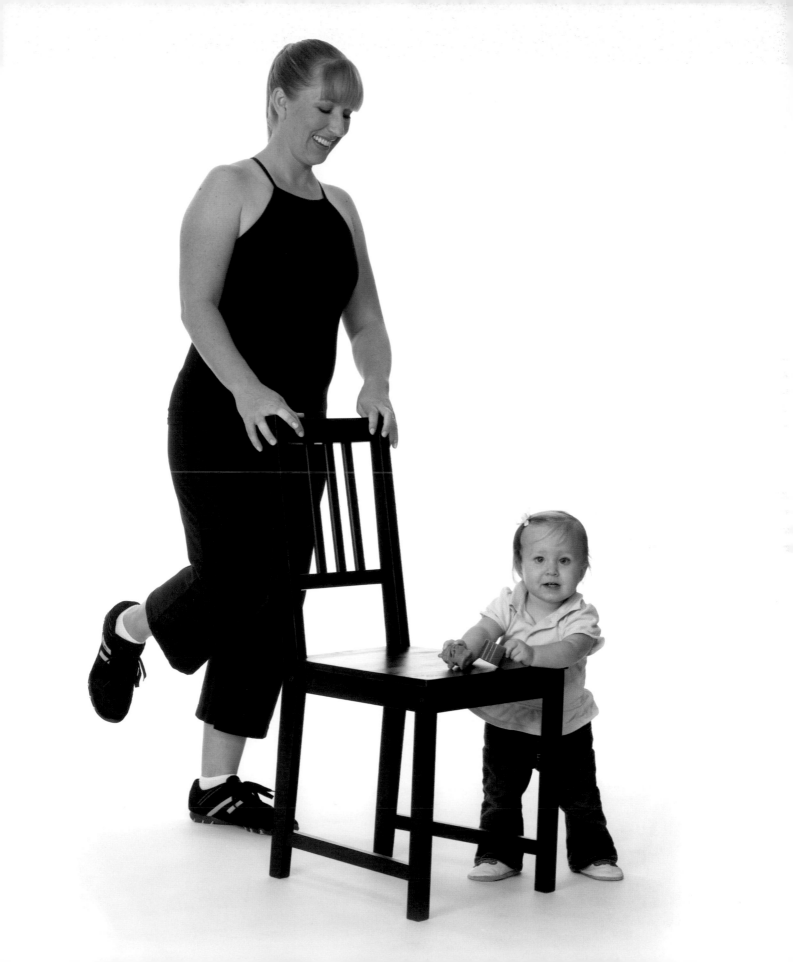

WHAT YOU'RE LIFTING THESE DAYS: YOUR BABY'S WEIGHT		
WEEKS	**WEIGHT**	**DATE**
44–45		
46–47		
48–49		
50–51		
52–53		
54–55		
56–57		

As your baby approaches her first birthday, her communication skills greatly improve. She may be speaking her first words already. Around this time, babies begin to understand simple instructions, such as "Give Mommy the ball, please." I've included a few ideas in this chapter (see the "Making It Work with Baby" tips) on how to foster your baby's language development while you exercise (how's that for multitasking?).

Finally, by this stage, you've got a baby who's in motion, whether she's rolling, crawling, standing up, or walking. You might have to factor in a few moments of chase-after-baby time per workout. But, hey, you'll also boost your overall calorie burn.

How to Get Started

The final two workouts here are the most intense compared to earlier chapters. Try Routine 1 for about three weeks. Then do Routine 2 for the next three weeks. After that, switch between this chapter's two nine-minute routines every three weeks until your baby is about a year old. From there, you can follow any of the routines in this book as long as you find them adequately challenging. Consider, also, adding new activities to your program, such as

end of this book, but my sincere hope is that you will continue on your path toward a lifetime of health and fitness.

What's Happening, Baby?

Nowadays, your baby—soon to be a toddler—may be pulling himself to a standing position using a low table, sofa, or even parts of your body as leverage. Don't be surprised if he tries to climb onto your back or cruise along your body as you perform floor exercises like the Abdominal Plank. With this in mind, take extra care to watch your baby's every move.

Every baby has different milestones within the first year of life. Some babies walk at ten months; some don't take their first steps until well after their first birthday. Don't fret if your baby isn't on par with the developmental markers in this or other chapters. They are simply meant as a guide to help you plan your workouts based on what your baby might be doing in each of your postnatal phases.

cycling, yoga/Pilates, or Baby Boot Camp classes. As with previous chapters, Routine 2 requires hand weights for resistance instead of your baby's weight.

You may repeat your workout a second or even third time (or do Routine 1 followed by Routine 2). Either way, you'll get a solid workout that lasts from about nine to twenty-seven minutes.

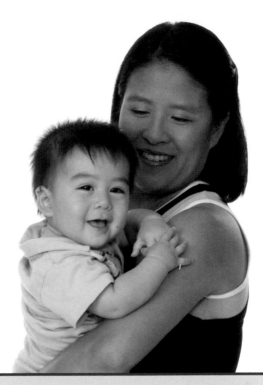

EXERCISE GUIDELINES FOR THIS CHAPTER

Read the steps below for what to expect from the workout in this chapter.

• Each strength exercise should last for about forty-five to sixty seconds. Lift heavy enough hand weights in Routine 2 (about eight to ten pounds [3.6–4.5kg]) to adequately challenge your muscles in the allotted time.

• For variety or more intensity, check out the Intensity Boost tips in Routine 1.

• Do one or more of the nine-minute routines in this chapter three to four times a week.

• Your baby may be too heavy these days for you to incorporate her as added resistance for certain exercises. Check out "Making It Work with Baby" for ways to keep your baby happy if you're not holding her.

• Follow the sixty-minute cardio workout at the end of this chapter. Turn to chapter 7 for postexercise stretches.

Stationary Lunges and V-Steps

Do it for: three minutes total

Minute 1:
Marching/walking

March on the spot or—if your baby is mobile—get warmed up by chasing him as he takes off crawling or walking.

Minute 2:
Lunge and V-step, right leg leads

This phase of the warm-up requires you to take big steps backward and forward. Do the following:

1. Place your baby in a nearby position, making sure that she doesn't end up underfoot.

2. Stand with feet hip-width apart. Step your right leg behind you so you are on the ball of your foot with your heel up.

3. Slowly do a lunge by lowering your back (right) knee toward the floor; keep your front (left) knee in line with your ankle.

4. Bring your right leg back to the standing position.

5. Step your right foot forward and about forty-five degrees to the right; immediately step your left foot forward and about forty-five degrees to the left. Return both feet to a standing position.

6. Imagine stepping in a V-shaped pattern on the floor.

7. Return to the starting position and repeat the lunge movement, still leading with your right leg.

8. Add arm movements: Press your arms in front of you at chest height every time you lunge. During the V-step, pump your arms close to your sides (similar to how your arms look when you power-walk or jog without a stroller).

Minute 3:
Lunge and V-step, left leg leads

1. With feet hip-width apart, step your left leg behind you, keeping the heel up and balancing on the ball of your left foot. Do a lunge.

2. Bring your left leg back to the standing position.

3. Do a V-step, leading with your left foot first (see instructions in Minute 2 above).

4. Return to the starting position and repeat the lunge, leading with your left leg.

5. Add arms movements: As you lunge, lift your arms to the sides, raising your hands to just below shoulder height. Pump your arms during the V-step (see instructions in Minute 2 above).

Crossover Stationary Lunges

Works: legs, butt

Making It Work with Baby: This movement requires balance, so you may need to steady yourself with a wall or a chair if you feel too wobbly (but work up to doing the exercise sans support). Besides, your baby may be too heavy to hold during this move and/or he might not have the patience to be held right now if he's on the go. Let him explore close by, or prop him in a stroller, high chair, or activity chair. Do the lunges right in front of him.

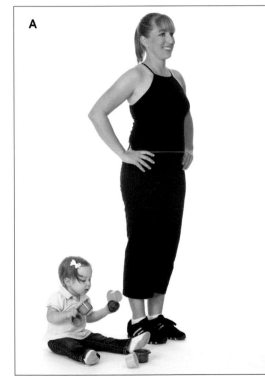

A. Stand with your feet close together.

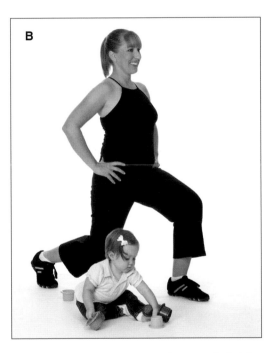

🌸 TRAINER TIP

Your back foot should be behind you but slightly to either the right or left (depending on your lead leg) of the front foot, which remains stationary.

B. Step your right foot behind you and slightly to your left, as you bend the back (right) knee toward the floor at the same time. This movement looks similar to a curtsy.

Return to the starting position. Repeat, still leading with your right leg.

Do crossover lunges with your right leg moving backward for twenty to thirty seconds, and then switch sides for another twenty to thirty seconds.

Plié-to-Squat Jumps

Works: thighs, butt

Making It Work with Baby: It's safest to keep a mobile baby well away from the "jump zone" during this move. A crawler could scoot from point A to point B at lightning speed, so secure your baby in a stroller, high chair, or activity chair during this move. Otherwise, it's OK to have a baby who's not mobile yet at a safe distance in front of you.

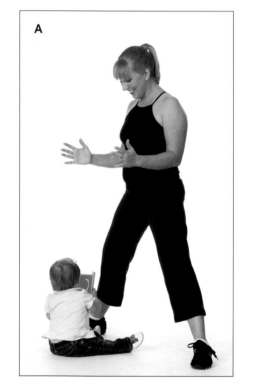

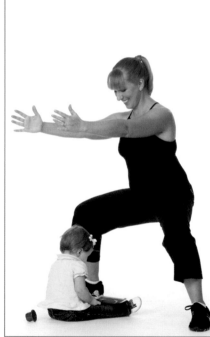

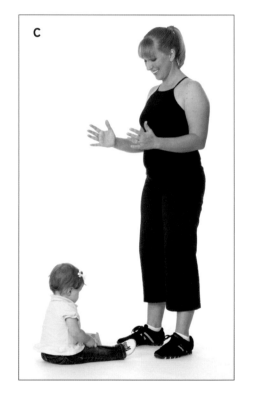

A. Stand with your feet wider than shoulder-width apart in a plié stance, toes turned out slightly. Bend your arms, keeping your elbows low and close to either side of your ribcage, palms in.

B. Do a plié-squat, extending your arms in front of you.

C. Once you've returned to standing, jump your feet together so they are about hip-width apart, toes pointing forward, as shown. Avoid rounding your back as you jump. From this position, bend your legs into a squat.

Return to standing. Jump feet to the sides so you are back in a plié stance. Repeat this sequence.

✿ TRAINER TIP
If you prefer to avoid high-impact movement, simply step your feet wide and narrow instead of jumping into those positions.

Wall Squats with Scapulae Squeeze

Works: thighs, butt, midback

Making It Work with Baby: Hold your baby close to your chest so she's looking outward. Count each squat as you lower to the floor, or recite "down" and "up" to help her get familiar with numbers and/or directions. If her extra weight makes this exercise too hard to do with good form for forty-five to sixty seconds, sit your baby on the floor by your feet.

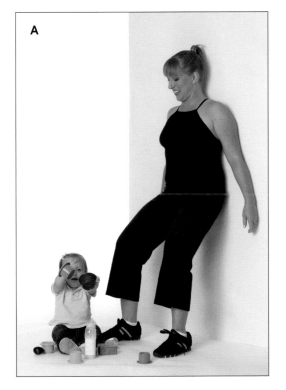

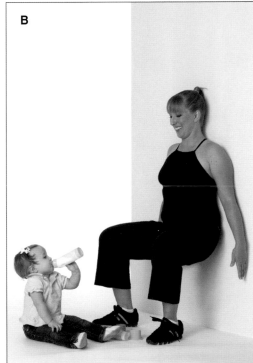

A. Stand with your back against a wall and your feet slightly farther from the wall than your knees. Draw your belly button toward the wall to engage your abs.

B. Slowly lower into a squat position, allowing your back to slide down the wall. At the same time, squeeze your shoulder blades (scapulae) toward each other, keeping your shoulders relaxed and away from your ears. Place your arms by your sides or hold your baby. Return to standing, release shoulder-blade squeeze, and repeat.

✿ TRAINER TIP

Place your feet far enough away from the wall so your knees don't push past your toes when you squat; keep your abs tight.

◎ INTENSITY BOOST

Lift your right heel off the floor so you are balancing on your left foot (which is flat against the floor) and your right toes. Do a one-legged squat with the left leg for twenty to thirty seconds; switch sides.

One-Legged Standing Calf Raises

Works: backs of lower legs

Making It Work with Baby: If your baby is too heavy to hold—facing either in or out—with one arm (and with good form), place her in her crib, on the floor, or somewhere where she's likely to stay entertained for the sixty seconds it takes you to complete this set.

🌸 TRAINER TIP

If you find it hard to maintain good balance on one foot, do these exercises with both feet on the floor.

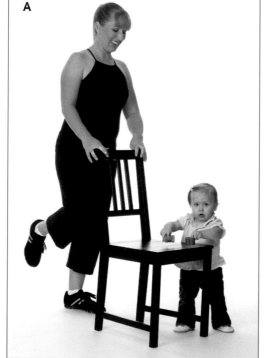

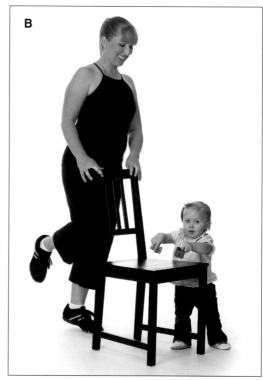

A. Stand next to a sturdy high-backed chair, wall, crib, or change-table to use as a balance support. Use one hand to support yourself.

B. Position your feet hip-width apart, and then lift your right foot off the floor, bending your right leg and holding your foot in the air behind your body. Raise your left heel off the floor and balance for one to two seconds on the ball of your left foot, as shown. Slowly return your left heel to the floor; repeat for thirty seconds. Switch sides.

Hands-to-Forearms Planks with Push-ups

Works: arms, shoulders, chest, abs, thighs

Making It Work with Baby: Place your baby between your hands, lying faceup so you can make eye contact with her. She may decide she'd prefer to be on the move, and, if so, proceed with caution: She may attempt to pull herself up using your body as leverage or even climb onto your back!

A. Lie facedown with your feet hip-width apart and your hands on the floor, slightly wider than shoulder-width apart. Your toes should be touching the floor with your legs straight and knees, hips, and chest off the floor. Engage your abdominals. Do one push-up.

B. Slowly bend one arm at a time to rest your forearms on the floor, elbows aligned under your shoulders, as shown. Return to the starting position by straightening your arms and placing your hands back on the floor. Repeat the sequence, doing a push-up every time you come back to the straight-arms starting position.

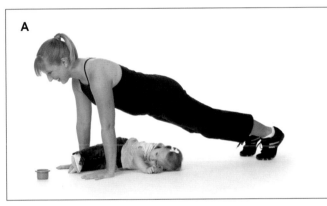

🌼 TRAINER TIP
Maintain a straight line from the back of your head to your heels. Don't allow your legs or stomach to touch the floor during your transition from forearms to straight arms.

◎ INTENSITY BOOST
Do one or both plank variations (on your hands and on your forearms) with one foot off the floor. Alternate between right and left sides.

One-Legged Bridges

Works: butt, back of thighs, lower back, abs

Making It Work with Baby: Your baby can sit straddled over your pelvis. Or, place your baby on the floor at your side with an arsenal of toys.

🏵 TRAINER TIP

Avoid letting your hips drop toward the floor— keep your hips up, reaching toward the ceiling. If this move feels too challenging, limit or eliminate the foot lifts.

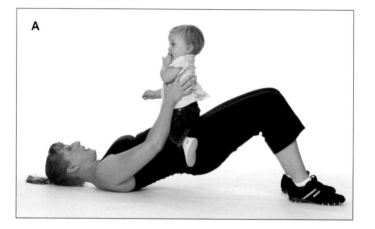

A. Lie faceup with your legs bent and the soles of your feet flat on the floor, heels about twelve inches (30.5cm) from your buttocks. Slowly raise your hips off the floor, squeezing your butt muscles and keeping your spine straight (not curving in or out). Your feet, shoulder blades, and head remain on the floor.

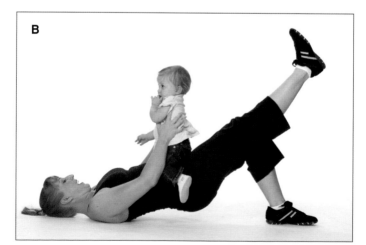

B. Lift your right foot off the floor and straighten your right leg in the air, as shown. Hold this one-legged bridge for three seconds before lowering your right foot back to the floor. Without lowering your hips, raise your left foot off the floor and hold for three seconds. Alternate between right and left foot lifts.

Abdominal Crunches

Works: abs

Making It Work with Baby: Your baby might like to sit straddled over your pelvis. Otherwise, try setting him on the floor beside you.

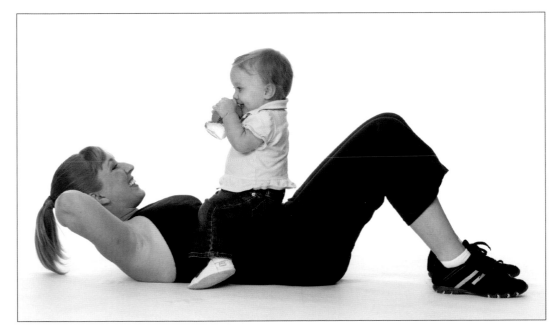

🎗 TRAINER TIP

To make the most of this exercise, imagine pulling the bottom of your ribcage to the top of your hips/pelvis each time you curl up. Avoid lifting your torso too high off the floor.

◎ INTENSITY BOOST

Straighten your arms and reach them over your head as you crunch (note that with this option you won't have a free hand to support your baby on your pelvis if needed).

Lie faceup with your knees bent, feet flat on the floor. Bend your arms, placing your right hand behind your head with your elbow pointing to your right side. Use your left hand to support your baby if needed (see "Making It Work with Baby"), or place your left hand on your lower abdominals to help you engage your deep ab muscles. Then curl your torso upward by lifting your head, shoulders, and shoulder blades off the floor. Release and repeat.

Low Back Extensions with Alternating Torso Rotations

Works: lower back

Making It Work with Baby: Protect your neck from strain by putting your baby on the floor to your right or left side instead of in front of you, where you'd have to crane your neck to see her.

TRAINER TIP

Rotate your torso instead of just turning your neck to the side. Keep your abdominals engaged throughout.

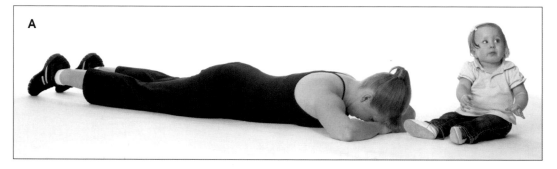

A. Lie facedown on the floor with your legs straight and shoelaces (top of feet) facing the floor. Bend your arms so your elbows point to the sides. Place your hands under your forehead, palms facing the floor.

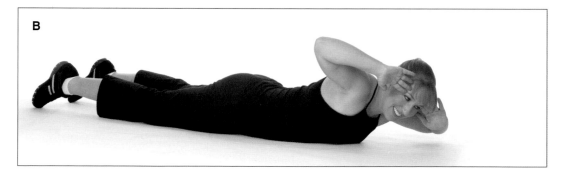

B. Gently lift your head and shoulders about three to four inches (7.5–10cm) off the floor. At the top of the lift, slowly rotate through your torso so your right shoulder (and underarm) faces to the right. Your right elbow should point up, and your left elbow may touch the floor. Rotate your torso back to the center position so you are once again facedown, looking at the floor, as shown.

Lower your upper body back to the floor. Repeat the sequence, rotating your left shoulder (and underarm) toward the left. Alternate sides.

Yoga Triceps Push-ups

Works: back of upper arms

Making It Work with Baby: Put your baby on the floor at your side with one or more toys to amuse him.

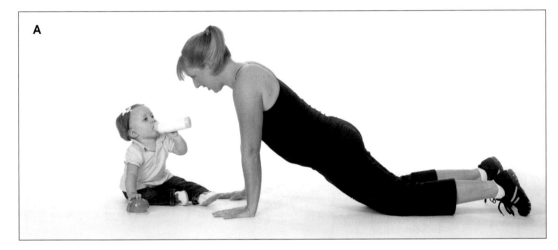

A. Get into a bent-leg push-up position with your knees and your hands on the floor, arms straight. Align your hands under your shoulders.

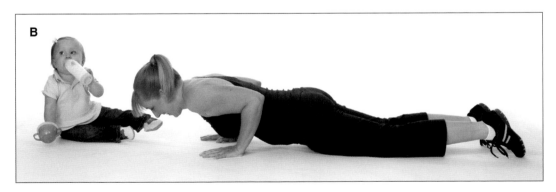

B. Bend your arms, bringing your chest toward the floor. Your upper arms should stay close to your body with your elbows pointing behind you, as shown. Return to the starting position. Repeat.

TRAINER TIP

Make sure your elbows keep pointing behind you (not to the sides). Avoid dropping your head as you lower into this triceps push-up— keep your face parallel to the floor and your neck in line with the rest of your spine.

Lunges with One-Arm Front Raises

Works: legs, butt, shoulders

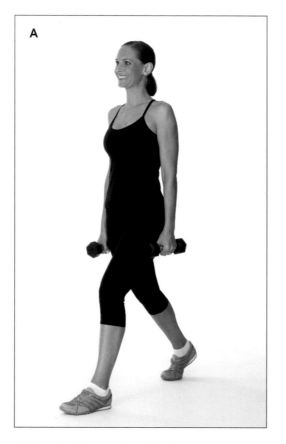

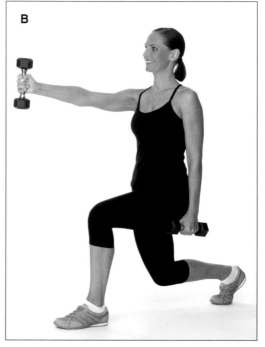

A. Stand with your feet hip-width apart as you hold the weights. Place your arms by your sides, palms facing toward your body. Step your right foot behind you and balance on the ball of your right foot. Your right heel should be off the floor.

B. As you lower your back (right) knee toward the floor into a lunge position, raise your right arm directly in front of you, palm facing in, thumb up. Stop the arm movement when your right hand is just below shoulder level. Your left arm remains at your side, as shown.

Lower your right arm as you return to the starting position. Repeat for thirty seconds, and then switch your working arm and leg.

One-Arm Reverse Shoulder Raises

Works: back of the shoulders

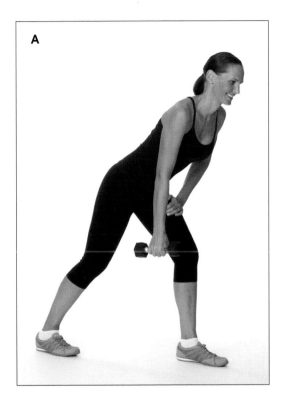

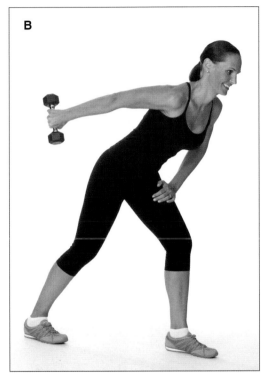

🌸 TRAINER TIP

Keep your neck in line with the rest of your spine and the working arm in line with your shoulder as you raise your arm behind you.

A. With feet hip-width apart and a weight in your right hand, step your right leg behind you, placing your heel on the floor, knee slightly bent. Bend your left (front) leg slightly and lightly place your left hand on your left thigh for support.

B. Bend forward from the waist, bringing your chest toward the floor without rounding your back. Your abs should be contracted. Hold your right arm straight, hand beside your right hip and palm facing your body. Raise your right arm about four to six inches (10–15cm) behind you, squeezing the back of your right shoulder, as shown.

Return the right arm to the starting position and repeat reps for thirty seconds before switching arm and leg.

Squats with Biceps Curls

Works: thighs, butt, front of upper arms

🌸 **TRAINER TIP**

Keep your elbows close to either side of your ribcage as you curl the hand weights toward your shoulders.

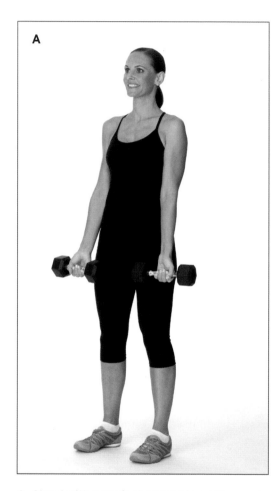

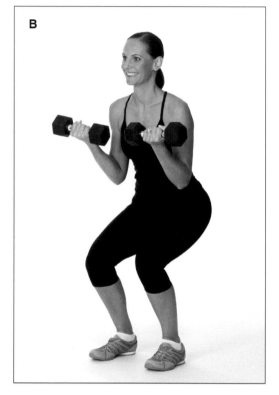

A. Stand with your feet about hip-width apart, toes pointing forward. Hold a hand weight in each hand, arms by your sides and palms facing forward.

B. Tighten your abs and slowly bend your legs, lowering yourself into a squat position until your knees are aligned over your ankles. As you squat, bend your arms, bringing your palms toward your shoulders, as shown. Return to standing and lower your arms so they are straight. Repeat.

Alternating Side Lunges

Works: thighs, butt, hips

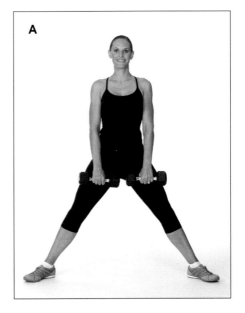

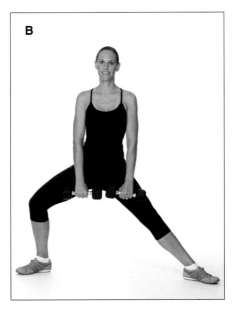

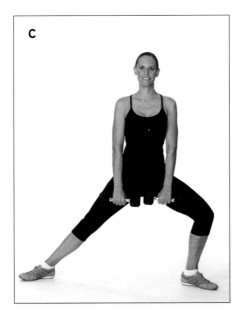

A. Hold a weight in each hand with your palms facing your body. Take a wide stance so your feet are wider than hip-width apart. Bend slightly forward from the waist, keeping your spine straight (not rounded).

B. Bend your right knee, lowering your hips toward the floor. Keep your left leg straight.

C. Push off your right foot to return to the wide stance. Repeat the side lunge by bending the left leg. Alternate between right and left side lunges.

🌸 TRAINER TIP

Stick your butt out behind you and keep your back flat as you perform the side lunge to ensure that your bent knee aligns over your ankle.

Deadlifts

Works: back, butt, backs of thighs

TRAINER TIP

Keep your abs tight, chest lifted, and back straight to avoid rounding your torso forward.

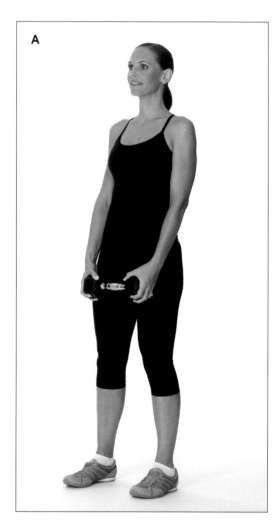

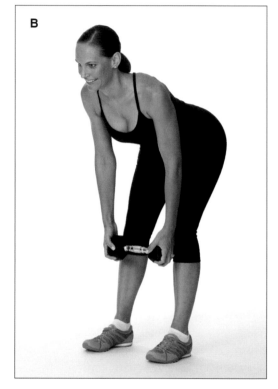

A. Stand with feet hip-width apart. Hold one heavy dumbbell with both hands and place your arms by your sides.

B. Engage your abs and lean forward from your waist, keeping your back straight (not rounded). Squeeze the muscles in your midback to draw your shoulder blades slightly toward each other. As you bring your chest parallel to the floor, allow your arms to hang in front of you with your hands in line with your shoulders. When you feel the muscles in the back of your thighs engage, pause, and then slowly return to standing. Repeat.

One-Arm Chest Presses

Works: chest, shoulders, arms, abs

A. Lie on your back with your legs bent and your feet flat on the floor, hip-width apart. Holding one weight in each hand, straighten your arms so your hands are aligned over your shoulders, palms facing your knees.

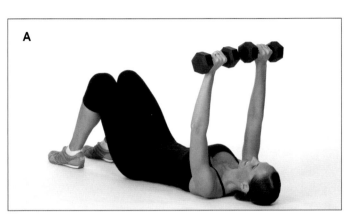

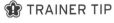 **TRAINER TIP**

Keep your lower spine close to (but not necessarily touching) the floor, instead of allowing it to arch up toward the ceiling.

B. Slowly bend just your right arm, lowering the weight until your upper arm is almost touching the floor. The knuckles on your right hand should be facing the ceiling.

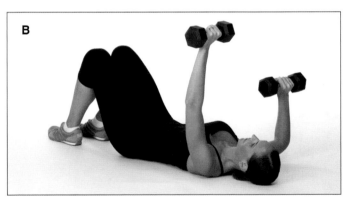

C. Slowly straighten your arm and repeat for thirty seconds. Switch to the left side.

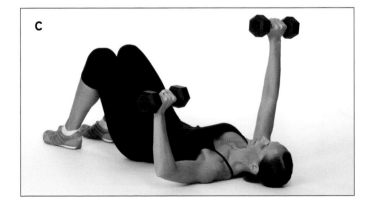

Straight-Arm Planks with Knee Drops

Works: abs, arms

TRAINER TIP
Keep your hips level so they don't tilt to the side as you lower your knee toward the floor.

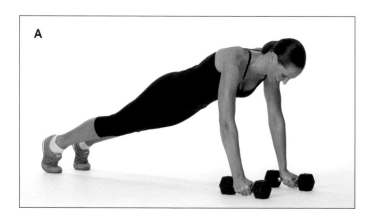

A. Place your weights on the floor beside you and get into a push-up position with your hands on the floor. Your hands should be aligned under your shoulders and your toes should be on the floor, legs straight.

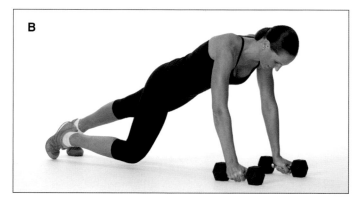

B. With your abs tight and spine straight (not curved), slowly lower your right knee toward the floor, keeping your left leg straight.

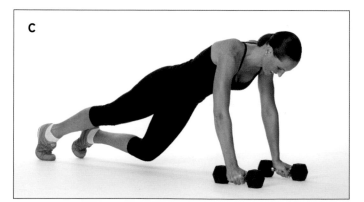

C. Return to the starting position and lower your left knee toward the floor, keeping your right leg straight. Alternate sides.

Abdominal-Crunch Presses

Works: front and sides of the abs, chest, shoulders

A. Lie faceup with your knees bent and your feet flat on the floor. Hold one hand weight with both hands, arms bent so you are tucking the weight toward your chest. Do an abdominal crunch, lifting your head and shoulders off the floor.

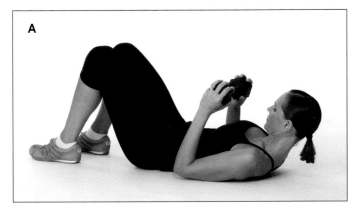

🏋 **TRAINER TIP**

Avoid tucking your chin into your chest or allowing your head to tilt backward—maintain a neutral position in your head and neck.

B. Then straighten your arms to press the weight toward your knees, as shown. Bring the weight back toward your chest before you return your head and shoulders to the floor. Repeat the sequence.

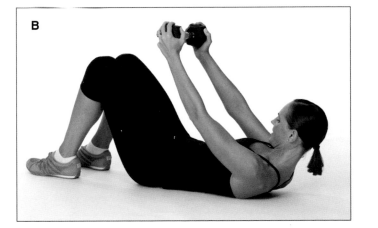

Supine Triceps Extensions

Works: back of the upper arms

TRAINER TIP

Keep your upper arms stable; your shoulders should not move during this exercise.

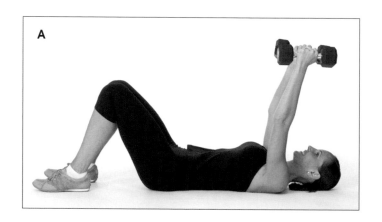

A. Lie faceup with your knees bent, feet flat on the floor. With a weight in each hand, straighten your arms in the air and align your elbows and hands over your shoulders. Your palms should be facing each other.

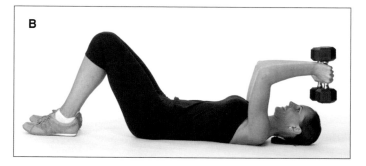

B. Slowly bend your arms, lowering just your weights toward your forehead. Keep your elbows pointing toward the ceiling and in line with your shoulders, as shown. Raise your hands to the starting position by straightening your arms. Repeat.

60-Minute Cardio Workout

Do this cardio workout four times a week with your baby in a stroller that you can jog or power-walk with. Check that you are at the right intensity with the

- "talk test" (you should be able to comfortably speak to your baby without gasping for air)

- the Rating of Perceived Exertion (RPE) chart on page 34

What You Need
- supportive shoes
- water bottle
- your baby in a jogging stroller
- a watch that shows time in seconds

Warm-Up

Do it for: four minutes

Start by walking at an easy pace, gradually speeding up to a brisk pace (RPE: 3). The warm-up should feel physically comfortable. You should be able to talk to your baby without losing your breath.

Drill 1: Six/Two-Minute Jog/Walk Intervals

Do it for: thirty-two minutes

Interval A: Jog (or power-walk if you prefer low impact) at a comfortable but challenging pace for six minutes. Each week, push yourself to cover a little more ground during this timed interval. Your RPE should be 6–7.

Interval B: Walk at an easy to moderate pace for two minutes. By the end of this interval, you should be able to speak comfortably to your baby. Your RPE should be 3.

Alternate Intervals A and B four times total (adds up to thirty-two minutes), and then try Drill 2.

Tip for walking with a jogging stroller: If your partner or another caregiver also takes your baby out in the stroller, readjust the handles back to your height before each workout (if applicable—not all strollers have adjustable handlebars). Proper handle height lessens the strain on your upper body and helps you make the most of every workout.

Drill 2: Two/Two-Minute Power-Walk Intervals

Do it for: twenty minutes

Interval C: Power-walk for two minutes at a challenging pace, taking long steps as you walk. Your breathing should be labored and you can only talk to your baby in short sentences. Your RPE should be 5.

Interval D: Switch to a challenging but moderately paced walk for two minutes. Your RPE should be 4.

Alternate Intervals C and D for five times total (adds up to twenty minutes).

Tip for jogging with a stroller: To make this workout harder, load the storage basket of your stroller with a few extra items (or, just don't toss out what's likely already in there—diapers, change of clothes, hats, blankets). To lighten the load and make the stroller slightly easier to push, empty the storage basket of nonessentials.

Cooldown

Do it for: four minutes

Walk slowly to cool down and allow your breathing to return to normal (RPE: 2–3).

Extending the Workout
After four to eight weeks: Squeeze in one to two non-stroller-walking cardio workouts per week (or as often as you can) to cross-train for injury prevention and faster results.

CHAPTER 7

Stretch It Out

In some ways, stretching is the unsung hero of fitness. I say that because exercisers at all levels typically overlook the crucial role flexibility plays in making you look and feel better. More often than not, people neglect stretching because they think cardio and strength training is all they need to achieve a nice-looking body and a better fitness level. Not so.

Remember in chapter 2 I discussed how pregnancy does a number on your posture? It makes some muscles loose and weak while others get tight and strong. Lengthening those tight, strong muscles with stretching improves posture (an important first step toward looking better). And it limbers you up so you feel good right away. Regular stretching also improves your fitness performance (helping you work out more efficiently), and it aids in preventing aches, pain, and/or injury.

If you're reading this soon after your baby was born, you might feel as if you're body's been put through the wringer. You're recovering from birthing a baby. You're sleep-deprived. You're catering to your newborn's nonstop needs. The last thing you need is uncomfortably tense, knotted-up muscles to slow you down. Good news: The simple and fast stretches (they last just ten to fifteen seconds) in this chapter will help you get through your day (and night) feeling less stressed and with fewer aches and pains. You can do these moves at home or on the go with your baby in a stroller. And on days when you don't have time for even a nine-minute strength routine, completing just a few of the stretches here will help you feel better and more energized.

To get started, simply read the Stretching Guidelines on the opposite page.

The following stretches are safe for all stages of postnatal exercise. If you are still recovering from delivery, skip any moves that cause you discomfort until your sore spots have healed.

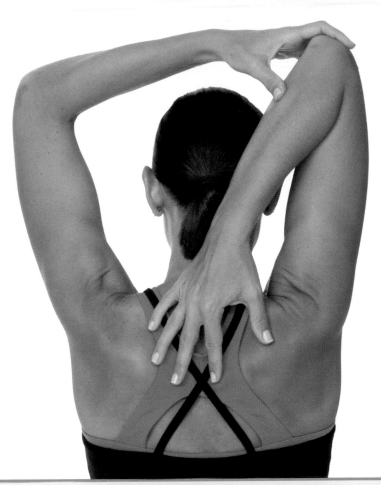

STRETCHING GUIDELINES

Do the stretches on the following pages after a strength or cardio workout, or as a stand-alone routine (warm up first, though). You can also squeeze one or more stretches into your day when you have a spare moment.

• Warm muscles stretch better and more safely than cold ones do. You may find that these stretches are more comfortable to do after a workout, a hot shower or bath, or when you've been chasing a mobile baby around.

• Even after pregnancy, your joints remain loose for about three months, or for as long as you breast-feed, due to the hormone relaxin. With that in mind, use extra caution to avoid overstretching. Doing the stretches here should feel good and relaxing, not painful or forced. Stretch in a controlled manner (i.e., not bouncing or

bobbing) just until you feel a mild tension in the targeted muscle(s).

• Breathe deeply as you stretch to help you—and your muscles—release tension.

• You'll want to de-stress and be able to hold these stretches without continually jumping up to chase a crawler or walker. If your little one's old enough to be on the move, wait until naptime for this routine or set him up in an activity chair, stroller, or high chair.

• Do the following stretches three to four times a week.

• Hold each stretch for ten to fifteen seconds (unless otherwise instructed in the descriptions that follow).

Standing Hamstring Stretch

Stretches: back of the thighs

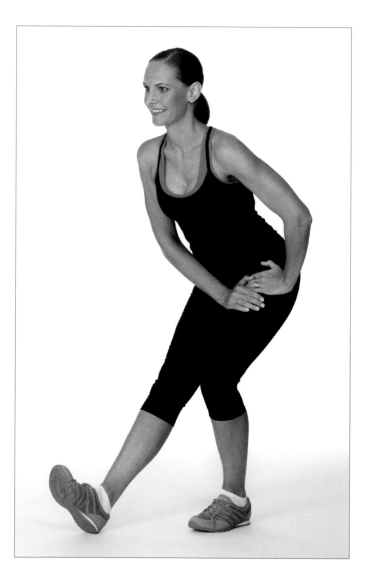

🌼 TRAINER TIP

To help target the right muscle group, imagine tilting your tailbone up toward the ceiling without overarching your back.

Stand with your feet hip-width apart. Flex the toes on your right foot toward you and place your right heel on the floor, a sturdy footrest, or a bench (if outdoors) slightly in front of you. With abs tight, lean forward from your waist, keeping your back straight. You may place both hands lightly on your left thigh for support. Return to standing and switch sides.

Standing Hip Flexor and Calf Stretch

stretches: front of the hips and back of the lower legs

From a standing position, step your right foot about twenty-four inches (61cm) behind you, toes facing forward. Press your right heel into the floor. Bend your left (front) leg, keeping your torso upright, chest facing forward, and your right (back) leg straight. Your back heel should remain on the floor. Return to the starting position. Switch sides.

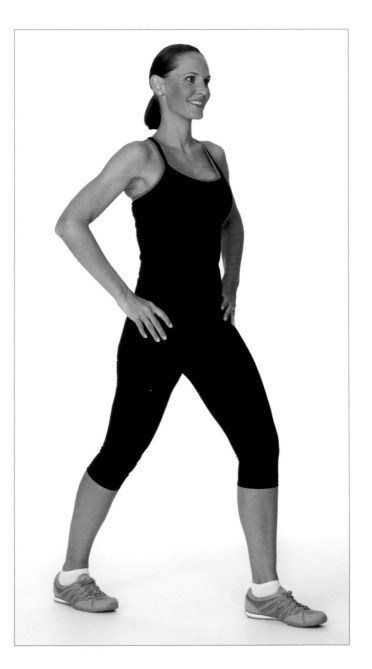

🏵 TRAINER TIP

Hold your abs tight to avoid arching your low back.

Standing Chest and Biceps Stretch

Stretches: chest, front of the shoulders, and front of the upper arms

TRAINER TIP

Avoid locking elbows when arms are extended.

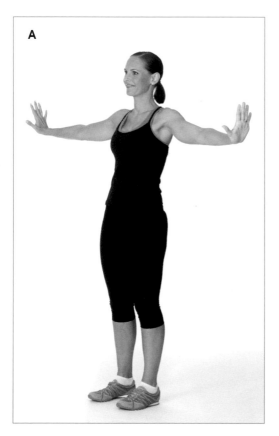

A

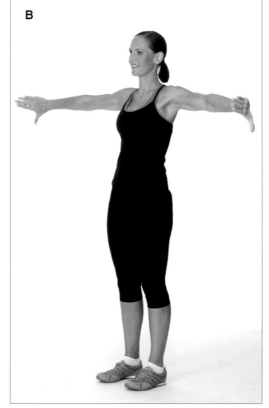

B

A. Extend both arms at shoulder height, pressing the heels of your hands as though you are pushing two walls away.

B. Slowly rotate your thumbs down toward the ground as you press your palms behind you slightly. Stop turning when you feel a gentle stretch in the muscles of your chest and shoulders.

Kneeling Back Stretch (Cat/Cow)

Stretches: low, middle, and upper back

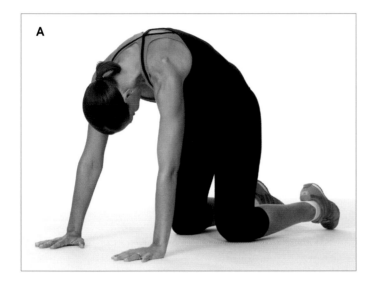

A. Kneel on all fours with your hands aligned under your shoulders and your knees aligned under your hips. Round your back, pulling your belly button up and in to create a C-curve in your spine (this is the "cat" stretch in yoga). Hold for five to ten seconds.

🌸 TRAINER TIP
To make the most of this exercise, allow your shoulder blades to move away from each other during the "cat" stretch. Gently contract the muscles in your midback to bring your shoulder blades slightly toward each other during the "cow" stretch.

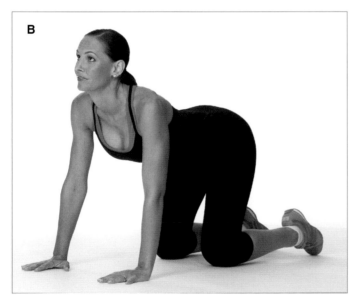

B. Now reverse the pose by gently arching your spine to create a small downward dip in your lower back while looking upward (this is the "cow" stretch in yoga). Hold for five to ten seconds. Repeat this sequence three to four times.

Side-Lying Quad Stretch

Stretches: front of the thighs

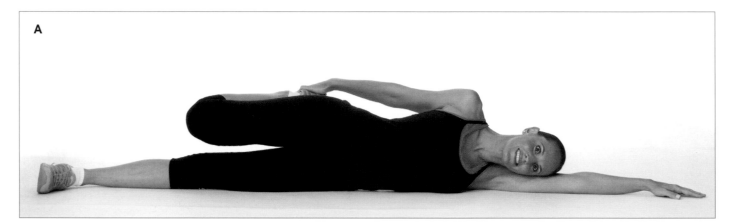

Lie on your left side with your hips and shoulders lined up. Extend your left (bottom) arm on the floor and rest your head on your arm. Then bend your right (top) leg so your right foot is behind you. Hold on to your right foot (near the shoelaces) with your left (top) hand, as shown. Switch sides so you are lying on your left side.

🌸 TRAINER TIP

Keep your knees side by side to avoid pulling your leg too far behind you.

Seated Gluteal and Hip Stretch

Stretches: butt and hips

Sit crossed-legged on the floor with your left foot closest to your body. Place your right (top) foot on your left knee. Then align your left (bottom) foot under your right knee, as shown. Draw your belly button toward your spine and bring your shoulder blades slightly toward each other. Lean forward from your waist to feel a deeper stretch. Switch sides.

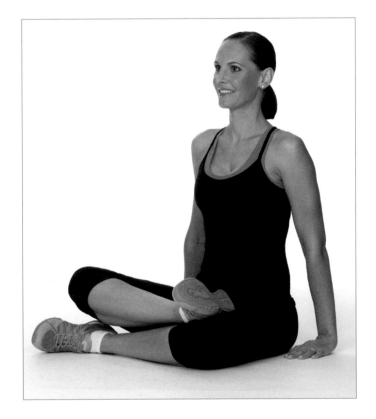

TRAINER TIP

If you feel discomfort in the ankle or knee of your top leg, align your top foot over your bottom calf instead of the bottom knee.

Seated Neck Stretch

Stretches: sides of the neck

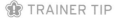 TRAINER TIP

Avoid slouching or forcing the stretch.

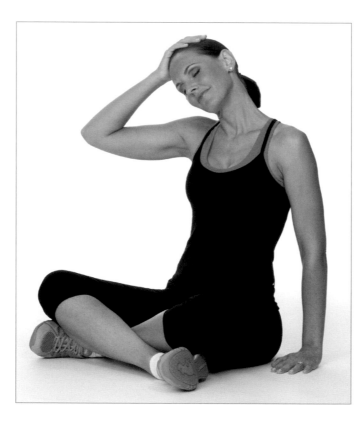

Sit comfortably on the floor or a bench (if outdoors). With your head in a neutral position (i.e., looking straight ahead), rest your left arm down by your side. Your arm should be straight with your palm gently pressing into the floor or a bench beside you. Gently tilt your head to bring your right ear toward your right shoulder. You can place your right hand on your head, applying gentle pressure, to help increase the stretch. Release and switch sides.

Seated Triceps Stretch

Stretches: back of the upper arms

Sit tall on the floor or a bench (if outdoors). Raise your right arm above your head, and then bend the right elbow, bringing your right hand behind your back, palm facing your body. Then place your left hand on your right elbow, gently pressing your right arm back to intensify the stretch. Avoid dropping your chin toward your chest. Switch sides.

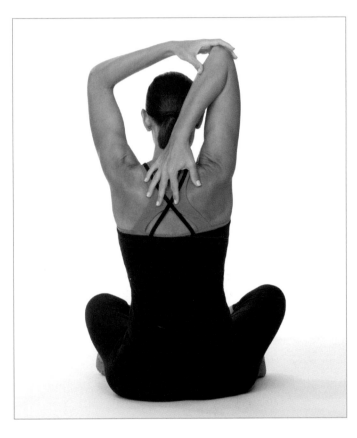

🌸 TRAINER TIP

Envision lowering the fingertips on your stretching arm toward your tailbone.

Seated Shoulder Stretch

Stretches: middle and back of the shoulders

🌸 TRAINER TIP

Keep your stretching shoulder down and away from your ear.

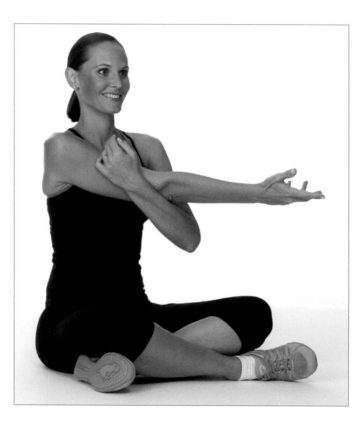

Sit tall and bring your right arm across your chest, palm facing behind you, thumb up. Then place your left hand on either your right forearm or just above your right elbow. Gently press your right arm toward your body to intensify the stretch. Switch sides.

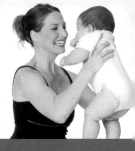

PART 3

Expanding Your Exercise Horizons

CHAPTER 8

Partner Exercises: Bonding with Baby and Friends

If you're used to leaving the house every day for work, you might be feeling as if sticking close to home with baby is quite an adjustment. Lots of moms find it downright lonely to spend so much time without their usual dose of adult interaction.

Let's face it. As much as you love your little one, there's no denying that, at times, caring for a baby or toddler (or both at once) can feel isolating, mind-numbing, and nerve-wracking. What mom hasn't felt a tad (OK, more than a tad) overwhelmed about her new life with such a precious but utterly dependent infant? Sometimes, it helps a whole lot to be able to vent or have a supportive shoulder to cry on—whether it be your partner's, a dear old friend's, or that of another mom who's facing the same elations and challenges as you.

Part of Baby Boot Camp's core philosophy is to foster social interaction between moms with babies and young children. We encourage women to make connections and share experiences with each other because, as moms ourselves, we know you need that kind of adult interaction to stay sane on some days! That's why I've included a partner exercise chapter in this book —consider it your excuse to call up a friend for comfort, companionship, and a workout. Partner exercise is a big trend in fitness right now, and it's the perfect solution to getting in shape while getting much-needed social time for you and the new moms you know.

This chapter contains six partner exercises you can do with another mom and her baby, or your spouse, or even your baby's older sibling. Your partner doesn't have to be at exactly the same fitness level as you. Her baby doesn't have to be the same age as yours, either. However, you will have to coordinate exercise dates that work for both of you in terms of potentially different naptimes and/or feeding schedules. After that, you're ready to try the exercises on the following pages. Start by completing a warm-up from any of the workout chapters in Part II (chapters 3–6). And if you like, review my tips in chapter 1 for making the most of exercising with your baby.

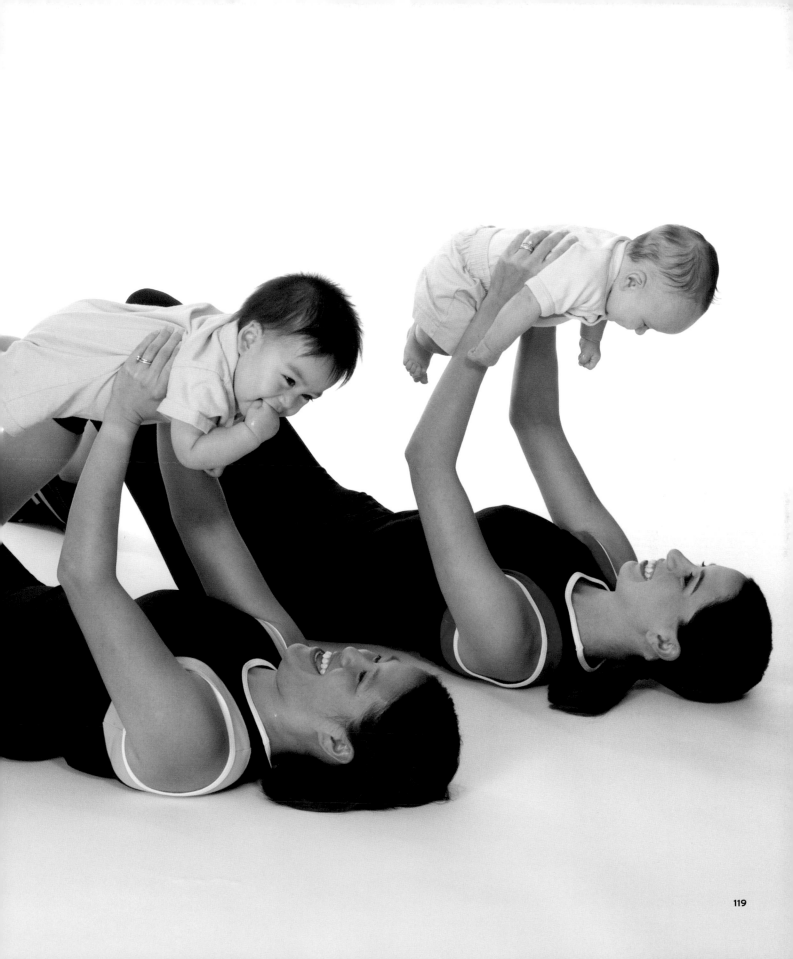

119

Partner Lunges

Works: legs, butt

Making It Work with Babies: You and your partner hold your respective babies in your arms or a front carrier. If possible, have the babies face each other. If your baby feels too heavy to complete this exercise for a full forty-five to sixty seconds on each side, place her on the floor or in a stroller or play chair.

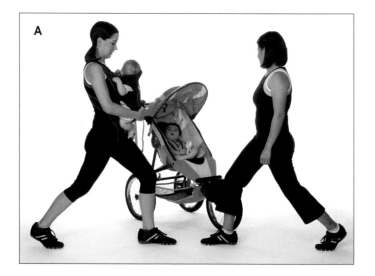

A. You and your partner stand facing each other with feet hip-width apart. Step your left foot behind you while your partner steps her right foot back so you are mirroring each other.

🌸 **TRAINER TIP**
It may be tempting to push your front knee forward, toward your partner, during these lunges, but to protect your knees and maintain good form, keep your front knee in line with your front ankle.

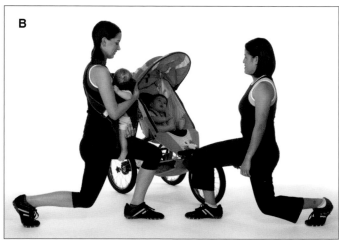

B. Lower your back knee to the floor to perform a lunge while your partner remains stationary, or perform the lunges at the same time, as shown. When you return to standing, your partner does a lunge, lowering her back knee to the floor, while you stay stationary. Alternate for forty-five to sixty seconds; switch legs.

Partner-Facing Plié Pulses

Works: thighs, butt

Making It Work with Babies: Have your babies facing each other as you hold them or wear them in a front carrier. Place older babies on the floor or in a stroller or play chair if you wish.

Stand facing your partner with your feet wider than hip-width apart, toes turned out slightly. Your partner does the same. Both of you then slowly bend your knees, lowering yourselves toward the floor as you perform a plié-squat. Then, with your legs still bent and in unison with your partner, gently pulse (make small movements, up and down) for ten counts. Both of you return to standing and immediately do another plié, holding yourselves in the down position and pulsing for another ten counts.

Return to standing. Repeat the sequence for forty-five to sixty seconds.

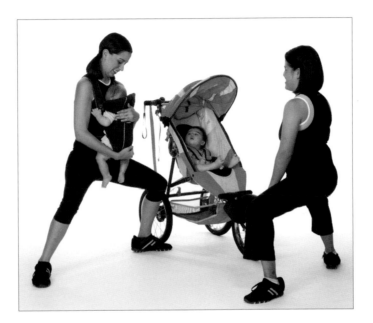

🏵 TRAINER TIP

If the pulsing motion fatigues your leg muscles well before forty-five to sixty seconds have elapsed, try plié-squats without the pulses.

Side-by-Side Baby Chest Presses

Works: chest, shoulders, arms

Making It Work with Babies: Hold your baby with both your hands under her armpits and around her torso, your palms facing each other. As you lift your baby, keep her aligned over your chest and look into her face. If your baby is too heavy to comfortably lift like this, try Kiss-Your-Baby Push-ups instead to work the same muscles (page 30).

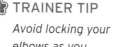

TRAINER TIP

Avoid locking your elbows as you straighten your arms.

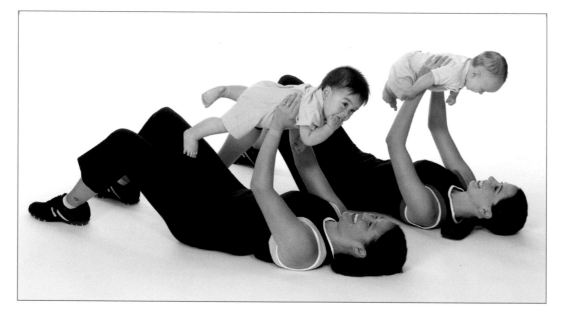

Lie faceup next to your partner. You should both be facing the same direction. Hold your babies so they are lying, tummy-time-style, on your chest. Tighten your abs and bend your legs, placing the soles of your feet flat on the floor for back support. You and your partner both gently lift your babies in the air until your arms are almost straight. Slowly bend your arms, returning babies to your chest.

Repeat for up to sixty seconds, depending on how long each baby enjoys this activity.

Rotating Partner Planks

Works: abs, back, shoulders

Making It Work with Babies: Place the babies on the ground or in strollers next to you. You should be facing either your baby or your partner and her baby with each rotation.

A. Lie facedown next to your partner with both of you in a plank position, arms straight and hands on the floor, shoulder-width apart. Hold for five seconds.

B. Rotate toward your partner so your bottom arm supports your body and your top arm extends toward the ceiling. Your partner rotates toward you, mirroring your position. Hold for five seconds. Return to a straight-arm plank. Hold for five seconds.

Reverse your direction so you and your partner rotate away from each other, following the instructions above but with the opposite arm supporting you. Hold for five seconds. Repeat the sequence for forty-five to sixty seconds.

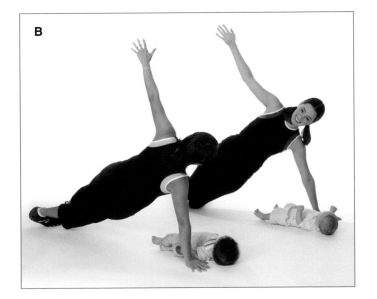

🏵 TRAINER TIP

To prevent stress on your lower back, avoid dropping your hips.

Rotating V-Sits (with ball or toy pass)

Works: waist, front, and sides of abs

Making It Work with Babies: Place babies on the floor by your feet so they can watch the two of you pass the object back and forth. You may also lean a small baby against your thighs, using one hand to support your baby and the other to pass the ball/toy.

TRAINER TIP

Keep your spine straight, abs tight, and chest open (avoid slouching or rounding the back and shoulders).

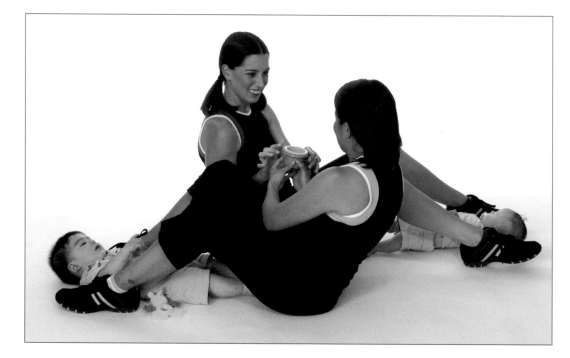

Your partner holds a child's ball or toy in both hands, arms bent. The two of you sit next to each other, hip to hip, but facing opposite directions. There should be about twelve to twenty-four inches (30.5–61cm) of floor space between you. Bend your legs, placing your heels on the floor in front of you.

Tighten your abs and slowly lean backward from your waist so the body forms a "V" shape from the top of your head to your bent knees. Use your abs to rotate your torso (avoid moving just your arms and shoulders) toward your partner as she rotates her torso toward you. As you rotate, your partner passes the ball or toy to you.

Return to the starting position and repeat, this time passing the ball or toy back to your partner. Continue the sequence for forty-five to sixty seconds, then switch positions so you each get a chance to rotate right and left.

Crab High-Five

Works: abs, back, shoulders, arms

Making It Work with Babies: Place the babies on the floor or in strollers by your feet so they can watch your movements from left to right and back again.

A. You and your partner sit next to each other with your legs bent to ninety degrees. You should be facing the same direction. Place your palms flat on the floor behind your hips. Your feet should be on the ground with your knees aligned over your ankles.

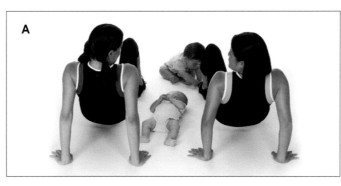

🛈 **TRAINER TIP**

If your wrists become fatigued, complete this exercise on your knuckles with straight wrists. Place a small folded towel under your knuckles for comfort.

B. Lift your hips off the floor and straighten your arms. Bend your elbows so they point behind you as you slowly lower your hips to the floor.

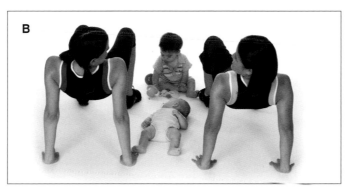

C. Return to the starting position. At the same time, raise the hand that's farthest from your partner's off the floor; she does the same thing. Make a high five in the air. Repeat the sequence for forty-five to sixty seconds; switch sides.

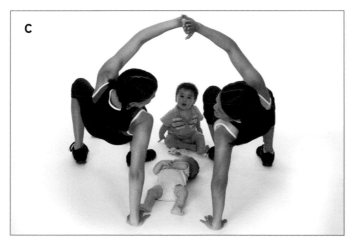

CHAPTER 9

Take It Outside!

I n the first few months of life with a newborn, you may feel as if you need to—and maybe even want to—stick close to home for the bulk of your workouts. With such frequent feedings and diaper changes, even a short trek outside may feel like a major accomplishment. Still, once you and your baby settle into a routine, there's no reason to limit exercise to indoors. You can make the outside world your gym, too. Exercise alfresco is a perfect way to have fun and get out of the house with your baby. You'll both benefit from the fresh air and natural light. For instance, even a brisk stroller jaunt around your neighborhood can lull your little one into a relaxed state and perk you up after an especially sleepless night.

So strap your baby into her stroller and load up on outdoor essentials. I recommend stashing the following items in your diaper bag or stroller basket for a safe, enjoyable workout outdoors:

• Diapers and wipes
• Blanket, pacifier (if needed), and toys
• Sun hat and sunscreen (depending on your locale and the season)
• Rain gear (depending on your locale and the season)

• A bottle and/or snacks for baby
• A water bottle and snack for you

After you've warmed up with five or more minutes of stroller-walking or light jogging, try the outdoor strength/cardio intervals in this chapter. This interval routine takes just nine minutes to complete (plus warm-up and cooldown). Interval training is a simple and efficient way to drop unwanted pounds and improve your fitness level. The reason: You're alternating between intense activity (which zaps lots of calories in a short span) and moderate activity (which lets you recover from the harder intervals while keeping your heart rate up). The only additional equipment you'll need is a sturdy park bench or a picnic table to get the kind of exercise variety that'll help fast-track your results.

When Your Baby Fusses in the Stroller

Exercising outside while your baby happily sits in her stroller is the ideal. However, in the real world, babies don't always sit still for our plans, do they? Your little one might be an early walker who prefers to hold your hand and amble alongside the stroller instead of riding in it. Or maybe she's prone to squirm and fuss when you strap her in

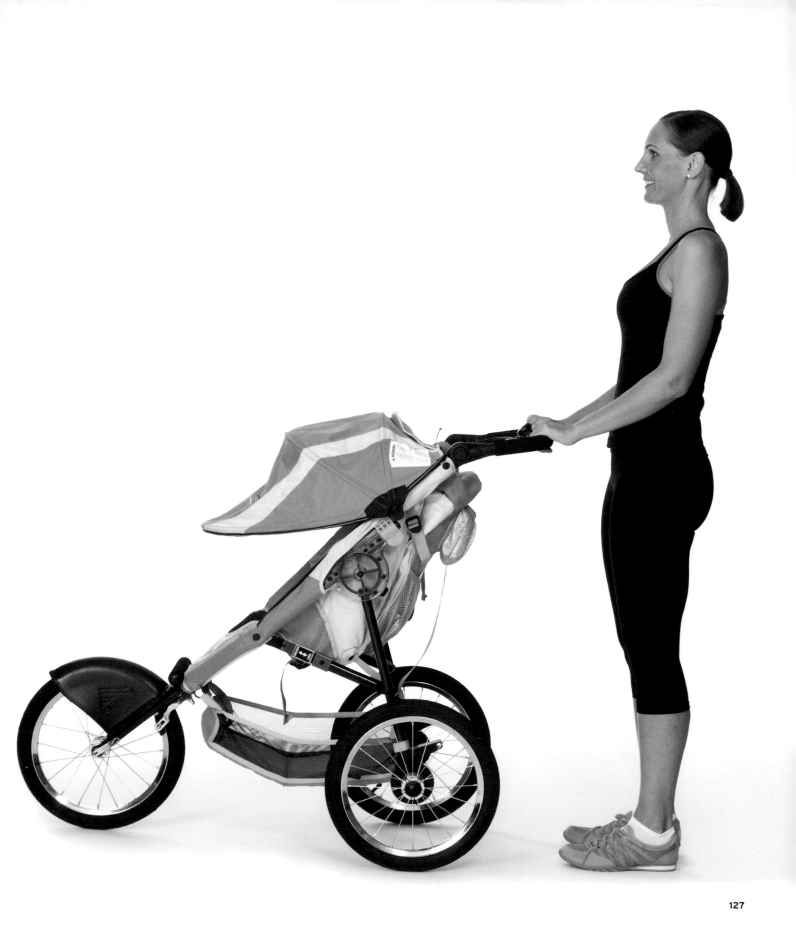

her stroller because she'd rather nuzzle close to you in a sling or front carrier.

How can you get a decent workout when your baby has other plans for how you'll spend your time outside? From my personal experience and from observing thousands of moms and their children in my Baby Boot Camp classes, I've come up with solutions that involve a combination of strategy, negotiation, and, yes, bribery. Read my tips below.

Talk It Out

Young toddlers understand much of what we say to them, even if their vocabulary level is too limited to reply. For example, while driving to my Baby Boot Camp classes, I used to discuss plans for the day with my young children. I'd say, "You'll get to see your friends at class and look for birds in the sky and puppies walking by. When Mommy is finished exercising, we'll have story time and we can go to the playground with our friends."

Time It Right

Getting a cardio workout outdoors with your child may require you to adjust the time of day you exercise to accommodate your child's nap schedule. While some babies are content to snuggle in the stroller with a blanket and let you do your thing while they snooze, others won't go down unless they're in their own crib. You know what works best for your little one, but be prepared for a possible shift in your baby's preference down the road.

From what I've observed in Baby Boot Camp classes, one optimal time to sneak in a cardio workout may be right after breakfast when your baby is well rested and fed (read: not cranky and only slightly impatient).

Use Bribery

I know, I know. All the parenting books tell us not to bribe our children. But when a meltdown is imminent and you just really want to get through all the intervals in this chapter . . . well, sometimes a bit of bribery is justified. Consider it your "Mommy needs her exercise to stay sane" line of defense.

Use a bottle to keep your baby happy. Or, if your baby is being breast-fed exclusively, feed him before you work out, then present him with a special toy that he doesn't see at any other time.

For babies who've started on solid food, offer healthy snacks (e.g., soft whole-grain or cheesy crackers, chopped up banana) using a special snack cup that they only get to use while riding in their stroller. Stocking the stroller with toys or books can also help stave off a full-fledged revolt. Sometimes the promise of a fun activity, such as feeding the ducks or a trip to the library can work, too.

Bottom line: Don't give up until you find something that works for you and your child. Remember, it's important for you to get your exercise, but it's also important for your child to witness your dedication to your mental and physical health.

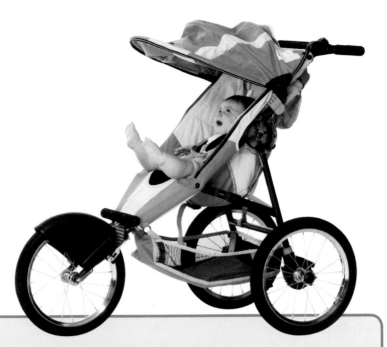

OUTDOOR INTERVAL WORKOUT

Follow the steps below for a time-saving outdoor strength and cardio workout. *Note: This workout is appropriate for women who are at least sixteen weeks postpartum.*

• Grab a stopwatch or wristwatch with a second hand so you can time your intervals.

• Strap your baby securely in the stroller and walk briskly or jog for at least five minutes to warm up. *Note: I recommend that you do not start jogging until you are at least four months postpartum.*

• Alternate sixty seconds of each strength exercise described on pages 130 to 134 with sixty seconds of jumping jacks, except the Hamstring Leg Extensions, which require thirty seconds per leg.

• Refer to the Rating of Perceived Exertion (RPE) chart in chapter 3 (page 34) for guidelines on working out at the right intensity. Your RPE for strength intervals in this chapter should be 4–6. Your RPE for the jumping jack intervals in this chapter should be 6–8.

• Cool down with gentle walking for two to three minutes. Squeeze your shoulder blades slightly toward each other as you push the stroller to work your upper and midback as you cool down.

• If your baby's mood is favorable, tack on as many stretches as you have time for at the end of your workout (see chapter 7).

Push-ups

Works: chest, shoulders, arms, abs

🌸 TRAINER TIPS

Push-ups: Avoid dropping your hips; maintain tight abs.

Jumping Jacks: Keep your knees slightly bent during each jumping jack. Nursing moms: Cross your arms over your chest if you need additional support.

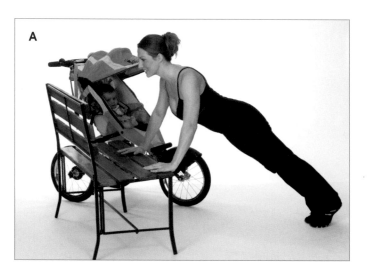

A. With your stroller beside you, place your hands wider than shoulder-width apart on a picnic table or bench. Your legs should be straight, with your toes touching the ground, feet hip-width apart. Note that your shoulders will not be directly aligned over your hands in the starting position.

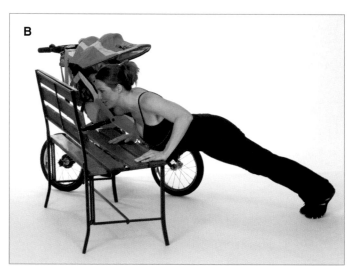

B. Tighten your abs as you bend your elbows to lower your chest toward the picnic table or bench. Your shoulders should be aligned over your hands in this position, as shown. Straighten your elbows, bringing yourself back to the starting position. Repeat for sixty seconds.

Jumping Jacks: Sixty Seconds

Works: cardiovascular system (heart, lungs)

Stand with your feet about shoulder-width apart, arms straight and at your sides. Face your baby. Jump feet wider than shoulder-width apart. At the same time, raise your arms overhead, elbows slightly bent. Return to the starting position; repeat.

Triceps Dips

Works: back of arms

A. Wheel your baby close to a bench or picnic table, facing you. Sit on the bench or the seat of a picnic table with the heels of your hands on either side of your hips near the seat's edge, fingertips pointing toward the ground. Your feet should be flat on the ground, knees aligned over your ankles, and thighs parallel to the ground.

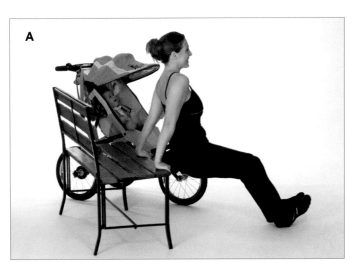

TRAINER TIP

Keep your elbows close to your sides and pointing behind you as you bend your arms.

B. Slide your butt off the seat but keep your hips close to the edge of the bench. Your shoulders should be in line with your hands. Bend your elbows to lower your hips just below the height of the seat/bench, as shown. Straighten your arms, bringing your hips back to the same level as the seat/bench. Repeat for sixty seconds without sitting back on the bench.

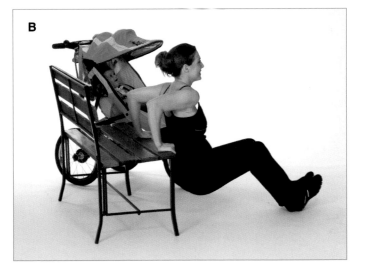

Jumping Jacks: Sixty Seconds

See instructions on facing page.

Alternating Reverse Lunges

Works: legs, butt

TRAINER TIP

You may be on uneven terrain in a park or playground. Before you begin this exercise, inspect the ground behind you for large rocks, holes, or sticks that could impede good form when you step backward.

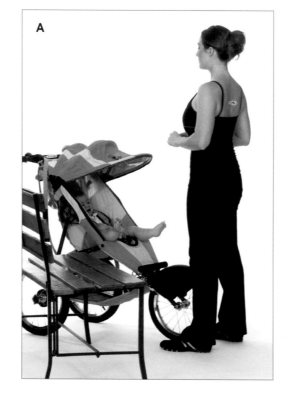

A. Stand with your feet hip-width apart so you are facing your baby.

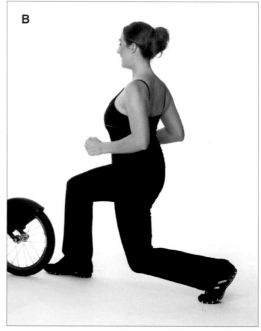

B. Step your left foot behind you and lower your left (back) knee to the ground. You should be on the ball of your left foot with your left heel off the ground.

Return to the starting position. Do a reverse lunge with your right foot stepping behind you as per the instructions in A. Alternate reverse lunges for sixty seconds.

Jumping Jacks: Sixty Seconds

See instructions on page 130.

Hamstring Leg Extensions

Works: butt, back of thighs

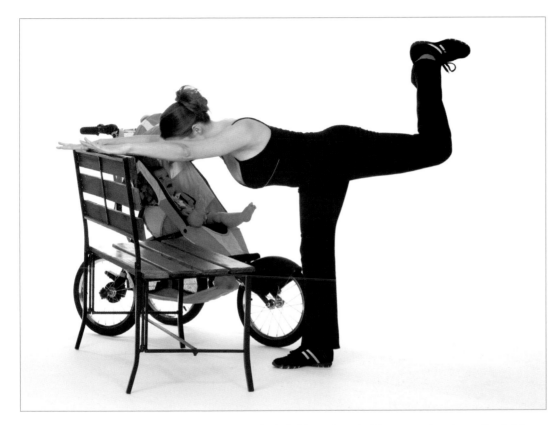

TRAINER TIP
Avoid tilting your pelvis to the side. Both hip bones should be facing the ground. Keep your abs tight.

With the stroller beside you, stand facing a picnic table or bench. Place your hands on the table or the back of the bench. (Alternatively, you can use your stroller handles—put the brake on first, though.) Lift your left leg off the ground. Keeping your spine straight, bend forward at the waist until your chest and left leg are parallel to the ground.

Next, bend your left leg to ninety degrees, so your left ankle is in line with your left knee and the sole of your foot is facing the sky. Pulse your raised leg (i.e., make small movements, up and down), pressing your raised heel about two to four inches (5–10cm) upward.

Continue the pulsing motion for thirty seconds. Switch legs and repeat for another thirty seconds.

Jumping Jacks: Sixty Seconds

See instructions on page 130.

Reverse Crunch V-Sits

Works: abs, back

Avoid rounding your shoulders or upper back forward.

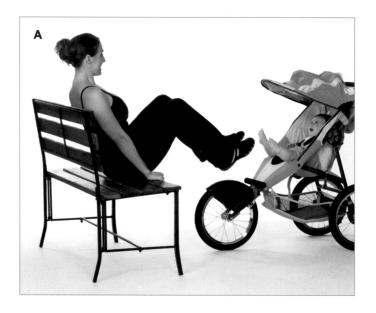

A. Sit on a bench or the seat of a picnic table facing your baby in the stroller. Place your hands on either side of you on the seat. Contract your abs and lean back slightly. Lift your feet off the ground and bend your legs to ninety degrees. Maintain tight abs and a straight spine as you slowly raise your knees about four inches (10cm) toward the sky.

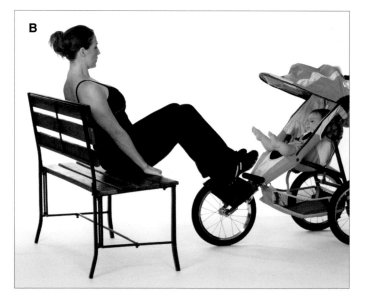

B. Lower your knees; repeat for sixty seconds.

Working Out with Two or More Kids

I've shown you how to do the exercises in this book with one baby. But, hey, that doesn't mean you can't successfully complete these routines with twins or even your baby and his or her older sibling(s). Here are tips for making your workouts work with two (or more) in tow.

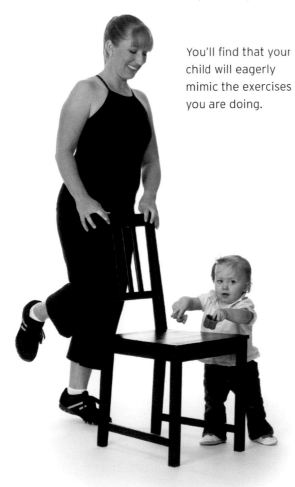

You'll find that your child will eagerly mimic the exercises you are doing.

Working Out with Twins

Alternate which baby you incorporate into the exercises. While you hold one, place the other in a car seat, cradle, stroller, or high chair (depending on the age of your babies).

Working Out with an Older Sibling

Toddlers and preschoolers love to join in, so encourage your child to playfully mimic the exercises you do (while you hold the baby). Make a game out of it. Children will, of course, do the moves with their own style—the point is to get them to be active and to keep them entertained alongside you.

Exercising Outdoors

A side-by-side double jogging stroller is best for two children or twins. Its wider wheel base makes it easier to turn, despite the extra weight you're pushing. As with any type of stroller, use correct body mechanics when you push. Refer to page 15 in chapter 2 to review the W.A.S.H. stroller posture.

Alternate your babies during the exercise routines.

On the Go with Baby in Tow

Choosing an Appropriate Stroller for Outdoor Physical Activity

Four-wheel, all-purpose strollers work well for running errands around town, but they're not great running (or jogging or power-walking) companions. Strollers that aren't designed for exercise don't handle the road well when you pick up your pace. Brisk walking creates too much friction on the stroller's wheels. And running or jogging with a regular stroller can be downright dangerous because your baby's "vehicle" wasn't designed for speedy maneuvers, quick turns, or a fast pace.

There are dozens of jogging, all-terrain, and off-road strollers on the market. Here are important factors to consider when buying and using a stroller for fitness.

Swivel-Wheel Strollers

The latest trend in strollers is the front swivel wheel. These all-terrain strollers were created specifically for urban shoppers and power-walkers, not runners. Many companies adapt the popular three-wheel style and market it as a "sport," "fitness," or "all-terrain" stroller. However, these "look-alike" strollers are not true jogging strollers because the twelve-inch (30.5cm) wheels are too small for a smooth push and ride at a jogging/running pace.

You can lock most swivel wheels in place, which is a good idea if you are jogging or running. However, if you intend to jog or do serious running with your stroller, opt for a true jogging stroller with three sixteen-inch or twenty-inch (40.5cm or 51cm) fixed wheels.

What *Is* a True "Jogging" Stroller?

True "jogging" strollers come with specific structural components. These include:
- three nonswivel wheels
- inflatable tires at least sixteen inches (40.5cm) in diameter (twenty-inch [51cm] wheels are recommended for more serious running)
- lightweight aluminum frame
- a hand brake for the front wheel, which helps you slow the pace
- a foot brake for the rear wheels to "park" the stroller
- an adjustable sun shade
- a five-point safety harness so your baby is securely strapped in
- a safety leash

Other desirable features to look for in a jogging stroller include:
- An adjustable-height handlebar. This is useful if you plan to share the stroller with your partner. An adjustable handlebar helps ensure correct stroller posture. It

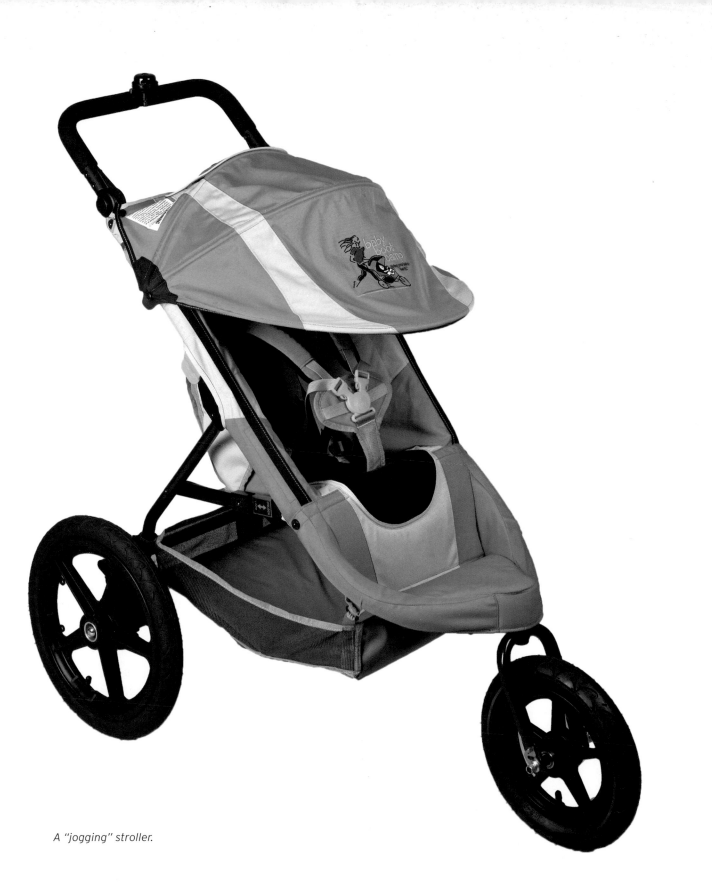

A "jogging" stroller.

also prevents wrist pain and discomfort for people with carpal tunnel syndrome. Varying the handlebar height to match your workout—walking slow, power-walking, jogging, running on flat or rolling hills—increases your comfort level and performance when exercising on your own or during Baby Boot Camp's stroller fitness classes.

- Reclining seat. If your child is less than six months old or has weak neck muscles, a reclining seat helps prevent the baby's head from rolling forward. It's also a nice feature for kiddos who fall asleep in the stroller.
- Under-the-seat storage bin. It's not essential, but it sure is handy for stashing workout gear and baby accoutrements.
- Safety features. Reflective fabric and/or an attachable blinking light on the stroller increase safety when you head out in the dark. Safety bells are handy when you're trying to pass someone with her iPod cranked.
- Comfort features—such as water bottle holders, key clips, and cell phone pouches—are nice perks.

Adjusting Your Handlebars
The photos show how to adjust your stroller's handlebars for walking and running speeds.

Determining Which Stroller to Buy
In the store, push every jogging stroller that meets your criteria. Once you narrow the field, test-drive the top contenders with your baby on board. Try out the stroller's brakes and folding mechanism for ease of use, and don't forget to check the stroller's dimensions to make sure it will fit in your vehicle.

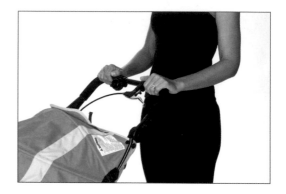

To adjust the stroller's handlebars for walking, set the handlebar height slightly above the height of your elbows to encourage proper walking posture.

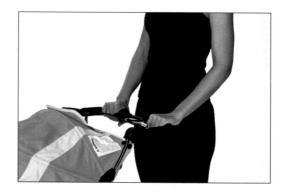

To adjust the stroller's handlebars for jogging or running, lower your handlebars just below the height of your elbows. This enables you to pivot easily when moving at a quick pace.

Every new parent loves a good deal on safe and functional baby gear. Although cost is definitely a factor in quality and durability, you can find a good jogging stroller for around $325 to $395. Jogging strollers that retail for around $150 are usually not as sturdy or long-lasting as those sporting a slightly higher price tag.

Acknowledgments

From Kristen

I'm excited to cross another thing off my list with the completion of this book. I could not have done it without an amazing support network.

My daughter, Madison, and my son, Tyler, were my true inspiration for developing the Baby Boot Camp program.

My husband, Mark, was the first to see my vision and help me to replicate and expand Baby Boot Camp beyond San Francisco. Thank you for always bringing out the best in me.

My parents, Dave and Carol, have always believed and supported me along the way. Thank you for helping me be confident in my abilities to do anything I wanted to do in life.

Thank you to the Baby Boot Camp Corporate Team for having as much passion about our program as I have and for supporting me each and every day.

Thank you to the Baby Boot Camp franchise owners and instructors who represent the Baby Boot Camp program in hundreds of communities by delivering safe and effective fitness classes for moms.

Thank you to all of the Baby Boot Camp students and my personal training clients who have encouraged me over the years to write this book.

Thank you to my literary agent, Laura Nolan, for believing in me and *Baby Boot Camp*. You stuck with us through so many life changes, including relocating and having more babies.

Thank you to the team at Sterling, including Jennifer Williams, for making this book a reality.

Last, but certainly not least, thank you to Amanda Vogel, who took all my crazy ideas and put them down on paper for me. It has been a pleasure to get to know you over the years and I look forward to what the future will bring.

From Amanda

When I learned about the plan for a Baby Boot Camp book, I was seven months pregnant with my first child. I was looking forward to life with a baby, and now I was going to write a book about exercising with one, too! This book's conception, "birth," and delivery spanned from my third trimester to just before my firstborn turned three and a half years old. Looking back, it was a busy time to say the least, but it turned out to be the perfect time for me to write a book for new moms, because I was one.

Thank you to the Baby Boot Camp team, but most of all to Kristen Horler. Kristen, thanks for your endless expertise, cooperation, and professionalism. I am truly inspired by your story and the Baby Boot Camp philosophy. Kudos to you for so beautifully coordinating the photographs shown on these pages. They make this book extra special.

Thank you to my literary agent, Laura Nolan, at The Creative Culture for your patience, direction, and clearheaded advice. I am grateful for all you have taught me about the process of writing a book.

To everyone at Sterling: Thank you for your support in bringing this book to the public. Jennifer Williams: Your expert editing and suggestions have made the *Baby Boot Camp* book that much better.

To Scott and my sweet daughter, Eva: I appreciate you being so patient about accommodating a writer on deadline. Scott, thank you for your support, superb parenting, and help in caring for Eva as much as you do while I write. Eva's love and hugs-for-mommy especially inspire me.

To my mum and dad, Andrea and Leo, my family, and my best friend: Thank you for telling me you are proud of me—it instills the confidence to pursue lofty goals.

The Authors Would Like to Acknowledge:

Photography
Riku
RIKU+ANNA Photography
www.rikuanna.com

Apparel
Jordan Veatch-Goffi
Doce Vida Fitness Inc.
www.docevidafitness.com

Hair and Makeup
Gina Lamm & Kari Larsen
About Face Design Team
www.orlandomakeovers.com

Models
Jaimie Johnson
Angela & Konnor Harvey
Julie & Noah Brum
Julie Childers Henry & Tasman Henry
Allison Kummery & Keenan Kummery-Yamuk

Index

About Baby Boot Camp

I first started Baby Boot Camp to help moms enjoy the many benefits of getting—and staying fit—together. One of Baby Boot Camp's key goals is to provide safe and effective workouts for real moms. It's been my pleasure to share my proven and successful program in the form of a book. To find out more about the Baby Boot Camp program, franchise opportunities, or to locate a class in your area, please visit www.babybootcamp.com. I sincerely wish you and your family a lifetime of health and fitness!